P9-CJY-151

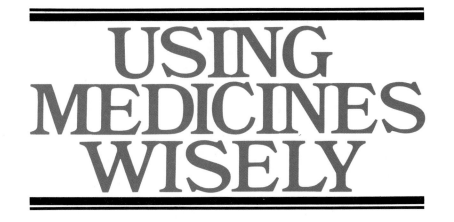

USING MEDICINES WISELY

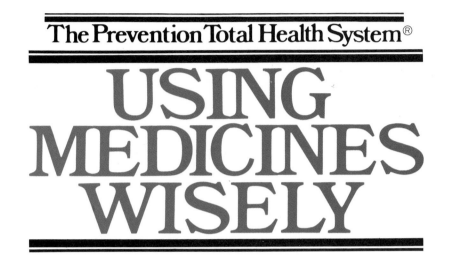

The Prevention Total Health System®

USING MEDICINES WISELY

by the Editors of
Prevention® Magazine

 Rodale Press, Emmaus, Pennsylvania

Copyright © 1985 by Rodale Press, Inc.

All rights reserved. No part of this publication may be reproduced or transmitted in any form or by any means, electronic or mechanical, including photocopy, recording, or any information storage and retrieval system, without the written permission of the publisher.

Printed in the United States of America on recycled paper containing a high percentage of de-inked fiber.

Library of Congress Cataloging in Publication Data
Main entry under title:

Using medicines wisely.

(The Prevention total health system)
Includes index.
1. Drugs—Popular works. 2. Chemotherapy.
I. Prevention (Emmaus, Pa.) II. Series.
[DNLM: 1. Drugs—popular works. 2. Drug Therapy—popular works. QV 55 U85]
RM301.15.U85 1985   615.5′8   85-2388
ISBN 0-87857-552-9   hardcover
   6 8 10 9 7 5   hardcover

NOTICE

This book is intended as a reference volume only, not as a medical manual or guide to self-treatment. If you suspect that you have a medical problem, we urge you to seek competent medical help. Keep in mind that nutritional and health needs vary from person to person, depending on age, sex, health status and total diet. The information here is intended to help you make informed decisions about your health, not as a substitute for any treatment that may have been prescribed by your doctor.

The Prevention Total Health System®

Series Editors: William Gottlieb, Mark Bricklin
Using Medicines Wisely Editor: Carol Keough
Writers: Stephen Williams (Chapters 1, 3); Gretchen Reynolds (Chapters 2, 9); Neal Fandek (Chapters 4, 7); Nona Cleland (Chapter 5); Mike McGrath (Chapter 6), with Debora Tkac, Neal Fandek, Denise Foley; Camille Cusumano (Chapter 8), with Neal Fandek, Stephen Williams
Research Chief: Carol Baldwin
Associate Research Chief, Prevention Health Books: Susan Nastasee
Assistant Research Chief, Prevention Health Books: Holly Clemson
Researchers: Tawna Clelan, Jill Polk, Carole Rapp, Martin Wood, Jan Eickmeier
Medical Consultant: Louis C. Lasagna, M.D.
Copy Editor: Jane Sherman
Copy Coordinator: Joann Williams
Series Art Director: Jerry O'Brien
Art Production Manager: Jane C. Knutila
Designers: Lynn Foulk, Alison Lee
Project Assistants: Lisa Gatti, Margot J. Weissman
Illustrators: Bascove, Susan Blubaugh, Susan Gray, Jerry O'Brien, Mary Anne Shea, Wendy Wray
Director of Photography: T. L. Gettings
Photo Editor: Margaret Skrovanek
Photographic Stylist: J. C. Vera
Photo Researcher: Donna Lewis
Staff Photographers: Alison Miksch, Margaret Skrovanek, Christie C. Tito
Production Manager: Jacob V. Lichty
Production Coordinator: Barbara A. Herman
Composite Typesetter: Brenda J. Kline
Production Administrator: Eileen Bauder
Office Personnel: Susan K. Lagler, Roberta Mulliner, Carol Petrakovich

Rodale Books, Inc.
Publisher: Richard M. Huttner
Senior Managing Editor: William H. Hylton
Copy Manager: Ann Snyder
Director of Marketing: Pat Corpora
Director of Book Production, Trade Sales and Subsidiary Rights: Ellen J. Greene

Rodale Press, Inc.
Chairman of the Board: Robert Rodale
President: Robert Teufel
Executive Vice President: Marshall Ackerman
Group Vice Presidents: Sanford Beldon
                       Mark Bricklin
Senior Vice President: John Haberern
Vice Presidents: John Griffin
                Richard M. Huttner
                James C. McCullagh
                David Widenmyer
Secretary: Anna Rodale

Contents

Preface

Drugs—Resources to Respect

One of the earliest memories I have—I must have been four or five years old—is of a sign plastered on the bricks of our row home in Philadelphia.

It said "QUARANTINED."

It meant I could no longer have my little pals come into our house and play. It meant a sense of dread for everyone in our family. It meant that my aunt, who lived with us, had contracted polio.

When they finally released her from the hospital, she looked frightfully pale and weak. Her left arm was paralyzed from the shoulder down and would never regain its strength.

It wasn't very long after that, that my parents marched all us kids to the doctor for the new—thank you, Dr. Salk!—polio vaccinations.

The conquest of polio is just one of many heroic victories by modern pharmacology. Searing infections, crushing mental illness, deadly metabolic disorders have all given ground to its power. Smallpox, just within the last few years, has been wiped from the face of the earth.

But pharmaceutical science had barely risen from its bows before it was dealt a smart smack across its face—with a royal glove, no less. "It is frightening," said England's Prince Charles not long ago, "how dependent on drugs we are all becoming and how easy it is for doctors to prescribe them as the universal panacea for our ills."

Ingratitude? Royal churlishness? Not really. Charles was voicing a concern that is felt today by millions of people—including, ironically, many physicians and other medical scientists.

It is commonplace now to hear experts on the benefits of drugs point out that antibiotics have been overprescribed for minor infections and even used for problems that don't respond to such treatment. Wasteful, yes, but worse: Yesterday's overkill is becoming today's underkill, as more and more strains of bacteria become resistant to overused antibiotics.

The overprescription and abuse of painkillers, tranquilizers and mood elevators has become not only a medical problem but a social problem as well, with astonishing numbers of people addicted to their chemical ups and downs.

Even the drug piled next to your pharmacist's cash register may have significant dangers, often unappreciated by their users. Nasal sprays, for instance, used for long periods, may cause a rebound effect that makes congestion worse, not better. Diet pills containing PPA are now under intense scrutiny because of their ability to produce sudden elevations of blood pressure.

We are now at the stage with pharmaceuticals where Stone Age man was after he first discovered that fire could be used to cook a goose, and then discovered *his* goose could be cooked by the same miraculous power. Like fire, drugs are neither friend nor foe. They are resources, and we must learn to use them with discretion.

Few of our resources, in fact, have the potential to help us—or hurt us—as much as drugs. Yet most people know remarkably little about them. After you read *Using Medicines Wisely*, which is part of The Prevention Total Health System,® you will be in an elite group. You'll be much better prepared to make good use of one of the most powerful tools ever discovered by the human mind.

Executive Editor, **Prevention**® Magazine

1

Total Victory in Two-Centu Is Proclaimed by Smallpox

By Victor Cohn
Washington Post Staff Writer

In 1796 a bold English doctor named Edward Jenner inoculated an 8-year-old boy with material from a cowpox sore on a milkmaid's hand. Two months later Jenner reinoculated the boy with matter from a human smallpox pustule.

Jenner called his successful new anti-smallpox technique "vaccination."

It took almost two centuries for the human race to fully apply it.

Today, however, billions of tragic cases of smallpox and billions of vaccinations later, the director-general of the World Health Organization will formally declare, "I personally believe smallpox has now been eradicated throughout the world."

If he is right—and it is two years since the last known natural occurrence of this once-global scourge—man has for the first time wiped out a major disease.

It was just two years ago today that Ali Maow ... ook in Merca, Somalia, was ... h a high fever and the ... WHO teams ... ht out

word—in 33 countries, including India, Pakistan, Indonesia, Brazil, Rhodesia and South Africa.

And a few generations ago, the sight of pockmarked faces, marked for life by this disease's deep scars, was still common in the United States.

"Smallpox has been called one of the most loathsome diseases," says Dr. Donald Henderson of Johns Hopkins University. "I know that no matter how many visits I made to smallpox wards filled with seriously ill and dying patients, I always came away shaken."

Henderson made many such visits. Now dean of the School of Hygiene and Public Health at Johns Hopkins, he led the World Health Organization's final campaign against the great killer and disfigurer. For a decade, until going to Hopkins in February 1977, he was chief medical officer of WHO's smallpox eradication campaign.

At the end of the campaign, when no more cases could be found despite great effort and a WHO offer of $1,000 for any report, he said, "We knew we had done it, but we couldn't believe it."

The campaign he supervised was highly sophisticated and intelligent.

In 1966, on a motion by the Soviet Union, the World Health Assembly, the representative body ...HO, voted to try to eliminate smallpox in

... has said, "I believe very ...

There ... effectiv... young ... Foege ... plies in

If w... not d... each k... and c... "sear... smal... the w... U.S.... T... ral ... a n...

THE N...

Link Between a Drug Taken by Pregna...

By ROBERT REINHOLD
Special to the New York Times

BOSTON, Dec. 20—A direct link between a rare but increasing form of vaginal and cervical cancer in young women and a hormone drug taken by their mothers during pregnancy has been confirmed by doctors here.

The doctors urge that physicians and parents carefully monitor the female offspring of women who had been given the drug, called stilbestrol,

area on the ... and their nomadic ...

out to be the site of smallpox ...

As recently as the summer of 19... more than two years ago, there were mor... than 2,500 cases in Somalia.

In the mid-1950s the disease was still ever-present—"endemic" is the public health doctors'

a synthetic estrogen that was banned recently by the Federal Government for use in pregnant women.

Stilbestrol had been widely prescribed since the nineteen-forties for women with a high risk of miscarriage until a team of doctors at Massachusetts General Hospital reported last year that they had traced eight cases of cancer to the drug.

Today the same doctors reported that a follow-up study had turned up 91 cases of the disease, called adenocarcinoma of the vagina, through-

out the United States and in three other countries.

Of the 66 cases for which maternal medical histories were available, stilbestrol was involved in 49 cases, and in nine others the mothers reported having taken some drug for bleeding or miscarriage but did not know what it was.

The disease is still relatively rare, known for many years. It is believed that hundreds of thousands of American women took the drug over the...

It i... areas like th... African rain forests a...

There was money: $96.5 ... tional funds, in addition to many natio... nal spending. U.S. money of course predominated ... ...uted directly, as well a...

last 2... ally do... ters un...

Becau... without s... discharge... by the so-c... T. Herbst, a g... recommend... tion. Althoug... it becomes far ... well to early tr... "We recomm... whose mother to...

Effort

rriors

strategies. Particularly
p devised in 1968 by a
h officer named William
a delay in delivery of sup-

everyone, said Foege, why
limited area surrounding
urned out that this "search
, inevitably known later as
" could effectively elimina
ations without vaccinat
n. Dr. Foege now direc
ease Control in Atlan
's last case was the l
mallpox, there has
—and two related

Swine Flu Shots Halted in Nation; Paralysis Is Cited

94 Cases of Syndrome Reported in 14 States

By LAWRENCE K. ALTMAN

Federal officials suspended the troubled nationwide swine flu immunization program yesterday
because of concern that the shots were possibly
linked to recently reported cases of paralysis.

Since the end of last week, the Federal Center for
Disease Control in Atlanta, which runs the nationwide immunization program, has been investigating reports from at least 14 states of 94 cases, four of
them fatal, of a form of paralysis called the Guillain-
Barré syndrome.

Federal epidemiologists said that they could neither prove nor disprove the possible connection
between the paralysis and the swine flu shots.

But to be on the safe side, Federal officials ordered
the program halted late yesterday afternoon.

Of the 94 reported cases of paralysis, 51, including the four deaths, involved persons who had received
ine flu shots between one and three weeks before
onset of paralytic symp

MES, THURSDAY, DECEMBER 21, 1972

omen and a Rare Cancer in Thei

e disease usu- ing pregnancy have a complete pel- published tomorrow in the New
their daugh- vic examination by her doctor after England Journal of Medicine. The th
often arises menarche" (the beginning of men- registry is supported by the Massa- de
is bleeding struation in puberty), Dr. Herbst said. chusetts division of the American
detected "If normal, we recommend this be Cancer Society and the National Can- that
r. Arthur repeated yearly, and more frequently cer Institute. only
he team, if abnormalities are found." The disease is thought to be the had be
amina- Along with Drs. Robert J. Kurman, first known example in which a to
thal if Poskanzer, Dr. Herbst and David C. carcinogen, or cancer-causing
onds a registry of the disease to which passes through the fetus in
hundreds of physicians have contrib
girl uted information. A revi
ur first 91 report

Miracles and Massacres

Drugs have saved millions and made millions. In the process they've also damaged the lives of many.

A pill for every ill. That's been the clarion call of pharmacists, physicians, illicit drug dealers, drug companies and psychiatrists for the last half of the century, and all of us at one time or another have answered the summons. There really is a pill for almost every ill. Those that haven't been discovered will be soon. There are pills that help you have babies and pills to prevent them, pills that will speed you up and pills that will slow you down—even pills that will do both at the same time. There are pills that make you grow hair and others that make you bald. You can take pills to lose weight or gain it, grow tall or not grow at all. You can even take a pill that will give you a tan while you sit inside.

Television advertises them, friends recommend them, investigators accuse them and public relations experts defend them, but with all this attention, how much do you really know about drugs?

Do you know, for instance, that some common over-the-counter drugs are dangerous when used improperly? That, according to the U.S. Food and Drug Administration (FDA), more than 600 prescription drugs on the market have almost no beneficial therapeutic effect?

Drug awareness will be essential for anyone seeking to stay healthy in the coming years. Pills for ills will become more complex. Frightening diseases will fall to the new compounds. But just being modern won't make these drugs safe. With all the regulations in the world, dangerous drugs are still released into the market. The drug world is complicated, with a past that's both checkered and glorious. The story of drug development will give you a healthy skepticism about drugs. It will keep you from blindly accepting what you are told. Read on. You've got plenty to gain if you learn and a lot to lose if you don't.

THE PHARMACEUTICAL INDUSTRY

The pharmaceutical industry is fiercely competitive, with high risks and the potential for enormous profits. Drug companies deal with people's lives: If a drug proves to be dangerous, like thalidomide, the company will suffer along with the patient. But if a drug proves to be a lifesaver, the company stands to rake in the cash.

Because the stakes are so high, competition among companies can reach almost absurd levels, prompting questionable behavior and newspaper headlines such as "Drug Battle Heats Up." Is it really a war? Judge for yourself.

- *Advertising Age* reports that two-thirds of drug companies' advertising budgets are spent on detail men—salesmen who tour hospitals and doctors' offices promoting their company's drugs and giving away free samples.
- Until recently, drug companies

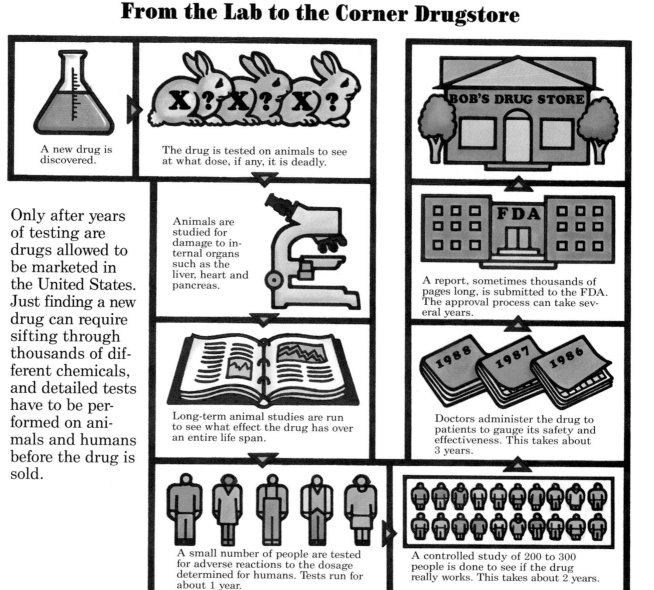

From the Lab to the Corner Drugstore

A new drug is discovered.

The drug is tested on animals to see at what dose, if any, it is deadly.

BOB'S DRUG STORE

Only after years of testing are drugs allowed to be marketed in the United States. Just finding a new drug can require sifting through thousands of different chemicals, and detailed tests have to be performed on animals and humans before the drug is sold.

Animals are studied for damage to internal organs such as the liver, heart and pancreas.

FDA

A report, sometimes thousands of pages long, is submitted to the FDA. The approval process can take several years.

Long-term animal studies are run to see what effect the drug has over an entire life span.

1988 1987 1986

Doctors administer the drug to patients to gauge its safety and effectiveness. This takes about 3 years.

A small number of people are tested for adverse reactions to the dosage determined for humans. Tests run for about 1 year.

A controlled study of 200 to 300 people is done to see if the drug really works. This takes about 2 years.

made a habit of offering high-priced gifts to physicians who frequently prescribed a certain drug. These included television sets, medical equipment and even upright freezers. Congress has since tried to ban the practice.

- An article in the *Wall Street Journal* reported that a physician recently made the rounds of television and radio talk shows in the United States to spread his message that it is dangerous to use generic (lower-cost, unadvertised) versions of prescription drugs when treating life-threatening diseases. What he didn't say was that the chemical makeup of generic drugs is identical to that of the name brands, but the generic drugs don't share the advertising costs. Another key point missing from his presentation was the fact that a major drug company about to face a challenge from generic manufacturers on one of its big-selling heart drugs was footing his bill.

- Drug companies routinely spend fortunes advertising their wares in medical journals. Doctors are supplied with preprinted prescription pads—preprinted with the name of the drug the company wants to sell.

- The quest for new drugs led drug companies to spend billions of dollars on research in the last 12 years. According to *Business Week*, double-digit budget increases have been approved for many research departments. In a recent year, Merck, Sharp & Dohme raised its budget 12 percent, to $400 million a year, and SmithKline Beckman Corporation's budget rose 10.7 percent, to $293 million. With the average cost of developing a new drug hovering at about $91 million, companies feel pressure to make back the money invested.

MONEY TALKS

The pharmaceutical industry is big. *Business Week* reports that prescrip-

Less Is Better for Mozambique

The revolution in Mozambique that led to independence in 1975 was long, difficult and anything but healthy for the soldiers and citizens caught in the crossfire. But it did provide an opportunity for the country to set up a unique health-care system—one that provides a good but sparse supply of drugs. You might think that good and sparse are contradictory words, but not to the people of Mozambique. Limiting the number of drugs used in the government health-care system to about 300 effective, inexpensive types has allowed the citizens of Mozambique to receive very good health care. All dangerous, unnecessary and nonsensical (because of outlandish price or exotic preparation) drugs have been replaced with standard-issue generic brands. Less-expensive forms of drugs—pills or powders instead of liquids and shots—are prescribed whenever possible. These are purchased on the world market through a competitive system of bidding that keeps the prices down. In addition, to prevent abuse, the government has devised a therapeutic guide that lists what drugs should be prescribed for specific illnesses.

tion drug sales alone totaled $31.9 billion in the world market in 1983. And the industry isn't slowing down. Prescription drug sales in the United States in that year were up 15 percent from 1982, to $15.6 billion.

In an attempt to justify spending $91 million in research on a single drug, most firms focus on developing drugs to treat common ills, and therefore drugs that will be used by many people. "Without a doubt, the prevalence of a disease is a motivating factor," says Jeff Warren, a Pharmaceutical Manufacturers' Association spokesperson. "Herpes is a good example. There is now a scramble to develop a drug to counter it." Yet sometimes the search for a drug to treat a common disease produces a surprise cure for a rare disorder. "It often happens that a company will come across a drug they weren't looking for that might apply to a lesser-known disease. The drug manufacturers have always developed these so-called orphan drugs that they come across," says Warren. "But sometimes university researchers will discover a useful drug and try to present it to the drug companies, who will sometimes ignore it because the cost of development is too high."

Fortunately, this problem has been alleviated, at least in part, by federal legislation that now gives drug companies tax deductions for the development costs of orphan drugs. And the pharmaceutical industry has created a commission on drugs and diseases to look at the feasibility of manufacturing the various orphan drugs that are proposed.

But the bottom line in drug development is . . . the bottom line.

Whether a drug is profitable or not matters little, however, to the people who must take it. Sometimes a drug can save a life or dramatically improve it. Sometimes it can destroy a life. What follows are the stories of some of the miracles and some of the massacres that have come out of the 20th century, the age of drugs.

ASPIRIN: FIRST OF THE MIRACLE DRUGS

One of the most remarkable drugs in use today is not usually thought of as being very special—it is just too common not to be taken for granted. But much like the sunset that occa-

Pharmaceutical companies spend great amounts of money developing drugs, but their investment pays off. The drug industry leads all others in the amount of return on sales. On average, for every dollar a pharmacy pays for drugs, the drug company makes almost 10½ cents profit.

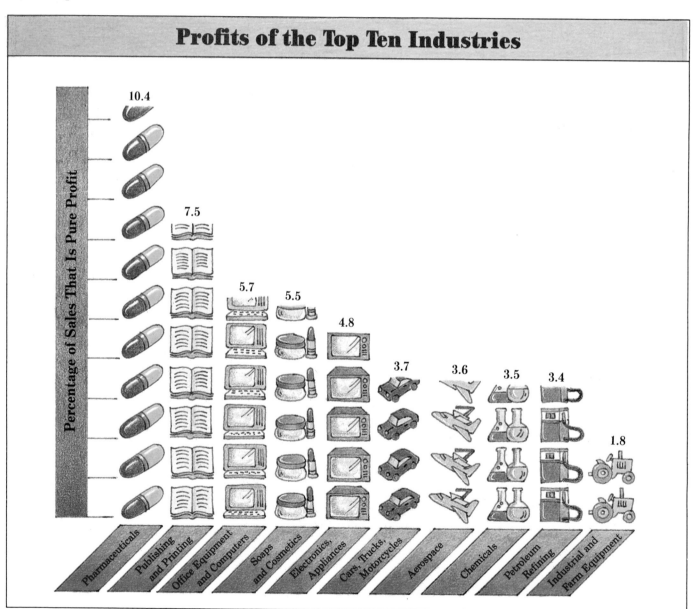

Profits of the Top Ten Industries

Percentage of Sales That Is Pure Profit

Pharmaceuticals	10.4
Publishing and Printing	7.5
Office Equipment and Computers	5.7
Soaps and Cosmetics	5.5
Electronics, Appliances	4.8
Cars, Trucks, Motorcycles	3.7
Aerospace	3.6
Chemicals	3.5
Petroleum Refining	3.4
Industrial and Farm Equipment	1.8

sionally astounds us even though it occurs each day, aspirin can be considered a miracle even though it accounts for one of the most frequently heard medical prescriptions: "Take two and call me in the morning."

Most times that morning call is a report of good news, because aspirin is surprisingly effective at quelling the pains of rheumatism, neuralgia, sciatica, neuritis and headache. And recent studies suggest that aspirin, because it is a potent anticoagulant (blood thinner), may help prevent heart attacks and strokes. And everyone knows how useful aspirin is for treating fever and inflammation.

With billions of doses sold in the United States each year (about as many doses as there are fish in the sea), a person who just found relief from a headache might wonder how anyone ever survived without the drug. What did the ancients do when the stresses of day-to-day life made them headachy and sore? Drink wine and race chariots?

Possibly, but they also took aspirin. Not aspirin as we use it—round tablets in plastic boxes or jars with childproof caps that are doubly difficult for adults—but aspirin in its natural form. The ancients chewed bark from willow trees, as did other groups throughout history, including American Indians. Willow bark contains salicin, a precursor of acetylsalicylic acid (or aspirin to all of us who never got around to taking chemistry courses in school).

Fortunately for us, scientists in the late 1800s devised a way to refine salicin, which can cause severe stomach irritation, to the more gentle compound acetylsalicylic acid. While high doses of modern aspirin can cause stomach upset, it remains one of the most beneficial modern drugs when used wisely.

FIGHTING POLIO'S DESTRUCTION

Polio is a word that burns in the American consciousness. Mention of it triggers a response in each of us.

All children born in the 1950s and later have the vague, almost hallucinatory memory of drinking red liquid from small, white, accordion-pleated paper cups, or of being frightened as the nurse prepared their arm for injection. It's a memory that blurs into the often-repeated "duck-and-cover" drills, black-and-white television broadcasts, hula hoops and Davy Crockett hats— just part of the way things were.

The parents of these children have different memories. They remember clearly the sporadic outbreaks of polio in the war years, when infantile paralysis, as polio was also called, would strike and not go away. Most diseases either leave their victims with no lasting reminders—or leave them dead. Polio, however, often left a telling emotional impression even on those it didn't strike. The sight of victims struggling in braces or lying in noisy, cold-looking iron lungs does not easily leave the mind. For years the only "treatment" for polio was to let the victim rest until the polio virus ran its course. The parents looked to the little cups of red liquid and the shots with wonder and hope.

Grandparents remember the 1916 epidemic in the northeastern states that hit 27,000 people, killing 6,000. The disease reduced New York City to a minimum-security prison, with passes required from people who wished to leave the city. Houses, blocks and whole neighborhoods were quarantined in what turned out to be a pointless effort to control the disease. Grandparents remember wondering where the horrible, crippling disease came from, and why it struck with such a vengeance.

THE POLIO PARADOX

The 1916 polio epidemic was one of the first in history. Yet polio isn't a new disease. Most experts agree that it has been around since civilization began, but never in the excruciatingly widespread and crippling form that appeared in 1916. Disease is usually associated with filth, but, paradoxically, polio became a problem in the United States when the country entered the age of indoor plumbing, sterilization and clean food.

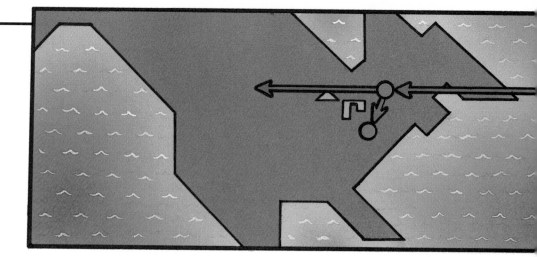

Polio is a disease that settles in the intestines. In the past, most people were exposed to the virus when they were young, because it spread quickly in the unsanitary conditions common everywhere until modern times. For various reasons, polio doesn't really hurt the very young, and when the disease struck them it passed harmlessly, leaving behind a lifelong immunity to further attacks. But with the advent of modern hygiene, fewer infants were exposed to polio. When they were a little older and finally did come in contact with the disease outside the home, they had no protection.

The fact that contracting polio prevented the disease from striking again was pivotal in developing a vaccine that eventually would conquer the disease. If polio virus is introduced to the body in a harmless dose, the body builds resistance. (This is the principle behind most vaccinations.) There are two types of polio vaccine, one made with live virus and the other with killed virus. The live type actually causes a mild case of polio that leaves the person immune without creating any serious side effects. The killed virus stimulates protective forces within the body as though the virus were active, again with no ill effects.

But neither vaccine had been developed when the National Foundation for Infantile Paralysis (later known simply as The Foundation) was established to help fight the disease which so many knew so little about. In 1940, it became The Foundation's goal to provide medical care for any polio victim who needed support. This private organization was embraced by Americans fearful of polio, who readily joined in The Foundation's now-famous "March of Dimes."

The Foundation amassed huge amounts of money from donors and set about reversing the ravages of polio. They found their guiding star in a restless and eager young man, Jonas Salk, M.D. Dr. Salk soon developed a vaccine, cultivated from polio virus grown on animal tissue, then killed. In 1953 he successfully vaccinated a small group of people. Encouraged by this test, Dr. Salk in 1954 conducted a trial with almost two million children, half of whom received the vaccine and half of whom didn't. There had never before been a test of this magnitude. For their contribution, the children were given a button designating them "polio pioneers."

While the early results of the test looked promising, the thorough analysis of the results needed to launch a full-scale vaccination program wouldn't be ready until it was too late to manufacture vaccine for the 1955 summer polio season. Yet if the results were positive, all of America would be clamoring for a dose and wondering why it wasn't available. Faced with the possibility of not having vaccine for the people who needed it, The Foundation gambled that the test results would be good and ordered 27 million doses at a cost of $9 million. This supply would either save America from polio or turn out to be a giant white elephant. A true mammoth.

Because The Foundation was privately funded, it had a strong desire for publicity, which might generate contributions. As the summer of 1955 drew near, the public

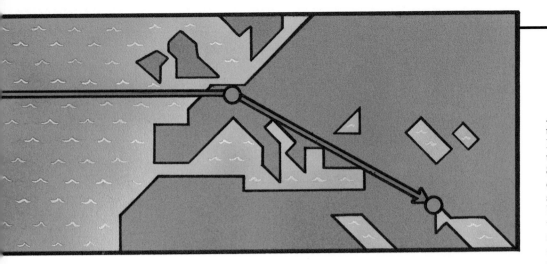

A surprise polio outbreak crossed the Atlantic to spread through Pennsylvania's Amish communities in 1979, seriously affecting 8 people. The reason: The Amish, distrustful of government intrusion and modern medicine, hadn't been vaccinated. Once convinced of the danger, most did submit to vaccination, and an epidemic was prevented. Surprisingly, the Amish polio got its start on the other side of the world, as the map shows. Virologists checked the virus's "fingerprints" and traced it to a Canadian strain that had been carried across the border by an Amish family. The Canadian strain in turn was traced to the Netherlands. And, say virologists, the virus might have originally come from the Middle Eastern country of Kuwait.

waited anxiously for results of the Salk test, and The Foundation devised a unique publicity stunt to announce the results. Instead of publishing the result in a medical journal, as was the usual procedure, The Foundation chose to trot out its findings at movie theaters around the country, so doctors everywhere could hear and see the results. The day they chose to announce the results "just happened" to be the tenth anniversary of the death of America's most famous polio victim, Franklin Roosevelt.

Of course, the announcement was positive. The test showed that the Salk vaccine, while not perfect, did work. Though the vaccine had actually caused a few cases of polio, it had prevented far more, and the wheels were set in motion for Dr. Salk's vaccine to be accepted throughout the nation. After a few setbacks, the Salk vaccine was seen as the polio savior, and Dr. Salk became a national hero.

SABIN'S WORK BEGINS

Most of America rejoiced, thinking the polio problem was over. Nevertheless, several scientists, most notably Albert B. Sabin, M.D., were working behind the scenes to develop a vaccine, made with live polio virus, that would be better than Dr. Salk's. They knew that Dr. Salk's vaccine was successful only if the patient returned for two follow-up shots— and, reflecting on human nature, scientists couldn't be sure of this follow-up. Moreover, no one knew how long the immunity would last. They also felt that a live vaccine,

because it could be administered orally and had to be taken only once for lifetime immunity, would be much more successful.

Dr. Sabin was convinced that this path was the chosen one, but few countries were willing to let him test his live vaccine on their citizens. Finally, he took his vaccine to the Soviet Union. On June 22, 1959, he announced that he had vaccinated 4.5 million people with no ill effects. At the same time it became apparent that Salk vaccine had caused—either directly or indirectly—204 polio cases, 11 of them fatal. The Soviets continued to administer the Sabin vaccine, but it wasn't until 1961, after 100 million people around the world had been vaccinated with no ill effects, that the U.S. began to seriously consider trading in Dr. Salk's method for Dr. Sabin's. Dr. Salk had saved the day in the previous few years, but clearly Dr. Sabin was the new hero. By 1962, the Sabin oral vaccine was the polio drug of choice in the United States.

THE MIRACULOUS MOLD

Penicillin easily upholds its position among the most remarkable drugs in use today. Since World War II, gonorrhea, syphilis, impetigo, strep throat, pneumonia, sinusitis, childbirth fever, lung abscesses and spinal meningitis have all bowed before penicillin's healing powers. Yet the drug—in its natural state derived from a mold much like the growth found on leftovers forgotten in the back of the refrigerator—has a his-

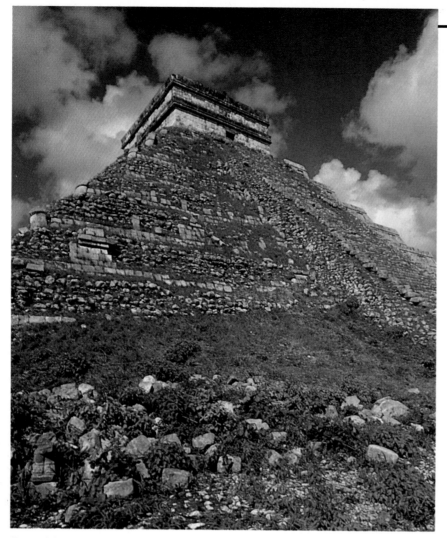

Ruins like this are all that remain of a great civilization ravaged by smallpox. In 1519, with the avowed intention of converting the "savages" of the New World to Catholicism, Hernando Cortez and 500 followers (mostly titled but landless Spaniards intent on establishing their credentials) arrived in Mexico. Though the Aztec leader Montezuma was initially friendly to the group, and even greeted them with their first taste of hot chocolate, Cortez felt it necessary to destroy this New World empire. Guns and horses helped, but the *primary* tool turned out to be disease—specifically smallpox, against which the Indians had no resistance. More than 3 million Aztecs died of smallpox as a result of Cortez and his merry men.

tory of neglect. Penicillin was discovered largely by accident and, once discovered, it was left to lie fallow for a dozen years before any practical way of using it was found. Still more years passed—with people wasting away needlessly from devastating infectious diseases—before the drug became widely available in the 1950s. Why the time gap? Penicillin came to scientific attention before there was a competitive drug industry such as now exists. Consequently, companies weren't willing to gamble time and money to make and sell this new drug.

Penicillin was first discovered in 1928 on a small petri dish of jelly in the dusty London lab of Sir Alexander Fleming, M.D. Legend holds that the penicillin mold entered the lab through an open window. This lucky event couldn't happen now, because modern laboratories are well-scrubbed—shiny and sterile enough to make a sanitation engineer smile—but Dr. Fleming's lab was of a

different age. One visitor said of it: " . . . trains hooted in the adjoining Paddington station and belched their smoke to blacken the laboratory windows and rush hour crowds swarmed noisily below . . . The laboratory was like a museum whose curator had died and the new one had not been appointed. There was labelled confusion. But there were no 'museum pieces' in that place; every specimen was working for its living. When the room became stuffy, windows had to be opened and all kinds of living dust invaded the laboratory to ruin the experiments, because the covers of beakers and the Petri dishes have to be removed sometimes."

SERENDIPITY

The story, perhaps romanticized over years of retelling, is that one day Dr. Fleming prepared cultures of staph bacteria for an upcoming experiment. He left the bacteria to multiply on jelly on covered petri dishes and didn't return to the lab for several days. Upon returning, he examined the dishes and saw that one cover hadn't been securely fastened, thus exposing the culture to invasion by impurities that drifted about on the London air. Instead of just tossing the mistake away, Dr. Fleming examined the mold and noticed that it seemed to be fighting off the infectious staph cultures. Whether or not he knew at the time the significance of the mold is a topic of hot debate. Although he was awarded a Nobel prize for his discovery, many scientists would characterize him as something of a bumbler. Nevertheless, the fact is that Dr. Fleming was looking at penicillin.

He apparently believed the mold would be useful for treating disease, but he wasn't impressed enough to vigorously promote his discovery. He did prove that the mold wasn't harmful by injecting it into healthy animals. But he didn't take the extra step of proving it was beneficial. Furthermore, he apparently made little effort to purify and concentrate the weak solution to make it more effective. Instead, he used it to treat external wounds, and had only limited success. When he found that his drug had a very short shelf life, he dropped the whole matter after a few unsuccessful attempts at preserving the penicillin.

While Dr. Fleming might be held negligent for not pursuing his work, at least he did make it public. Why didn't other researchers or drug companies investigate this compound that so successfully killed bacteria? First, scientists in the early 20th century didn't believe that a substance could selectively kill bacteria; they believed that the drug would also kill the cells in the body as it wiped out bacteria. To them it was like dropping a bomb on a civilian population in an attempt to kill scattered enemy soldiers. Second, most drug research was done by universities. While some companies made aspirin and even insulin, none had sophisticated research labs, so it would have been difficult for them to develop a new drug. And there was then no precedent for "miracle" drugs that would generate great profits while curing millions.

Paradoxically, it took the development of another class of drugs to change the way the scientists looked at bacteria-fighting drugs. The sulfa drugs, developed in the 1930s, proved to combat bacteria selectively, without interfering with other cells in the body. In other words, they didn't kill civilians along with the soldiers. Sulfa drugs became part of a new class called bacterial antagonists. The drug and chemical companies spotted the potential for profits, and the competition for synthesizing new sulfa compounds heated up as the companies began to develop their own research departments.

Spurred by the success of sulfa drugs, a group of scientists at Oxford University began in the late 1930s to investigate a broad range of bacterial antagonists. Though they had no intention of doing so at the time, the researchers, led by Lord Howard Florey, M.D., and Sir Ernst Chain, M.D., were to spearhead the mass production of penicillin and the resulting reduction in human misery and death.

The scientists were involved in a pure academic pursuit of knowledge about the bacterial antagonists. They weren't preoccupied with lust for a wonder drug. But Dr. Florey and Dr. Chain came across Dr. Fleming's earlier observations about penicillin while searching the literature about bacterial antagonists. Dr. Fleming had been stymied by penicillin's short shelf life, but Dr. Florey and Dr. Chain accidentally found that a form of freeze-dried penicillin was 20 times more active than even the strongest sulfa drugs—and it had a long shelf life, too. They tested the powder on mice: Four sick mice were treated and four were not, and only the treated mice survived. Clearly the scientists were on to something big.

HOPE FROM A FAILED TEST

The penicillin fungus was extremely difficult to cultivate in bulk. It took months to amass even a few grams. Bolstered by their experiments, the scientists decided to treat a policeman in whom a facial scratch had turned into a major infection. Such a serious infection would be rare now, of course, but at the time it was life-threatening. So, on February 12, 1941, C. M. Fletcher, M.D., of the Oxford group, began intravenous treatment with 4½ grams of penicillin that the doctors had painstakingly manufactured. It was, in fact, all the penicillin on earth. By the fourth day of treatment the policeman was eating and his fever had almost disappeared—a miracle for those days—but the penicillin was nearly gone. The man died ten days later because of this shortage. Still, his early improvement suggested that penicillin might be a great drug. Five more patients were treated soon after the policeman, and all were cured of their infections.

These recoveries caused the doctors to look for more efficient methods of manufacturing penicillin. These were war years, and Germany was spreading destruction across Europe; the scientists couldn't get proper laboratory equipment without diverting valuable materials from the war effort. So they had to rely on common objects to do the job: milk bottles, pie dishes, biscuit tins and even bedpans were used to grow

Smallpox Is (Not) Dead

The headlines read, "Smallpox Is Dead." But that wasn't quite the truth. The virus is alive in two labs, one in the Soviet Union, the other in Georgia at the Centers for Disease Control (CDC). Stanley Foster, M.D., of the CDC, says the virus is used by researchers to study types of pox. The World Health Organization now monitors both labs for safety, but precautions weren't always a major emphasis. In the 1970s, when other labs also kept the virus, it escaped confinement twice, causing minor outbreaks and even deaths in the U.K.

9

cultures. None of these worked well, but the scientists finally found potters in the north of England who were able to make special containers that did work.

WAR EFFORT DIVERTS SUPPLIES

Meanwhile, the scientists sought help from America, hoping the Yanks could provide penicillin for the British studies. A research center in Peoria, Illinois, developed a modern penicillin lab, raising the Oxford group's hopes. Then the Japanese bombed Pearl Harbor. Needless to say, the American-made penicillin was never sent to Oxford for further study—it went instead to the American war effort. With the war at full steam, the race for better penicillin picked up. New strains of the mold were found—strains that produced better yields of the drug. Penicillin manufacture rapidly became big business.

WIPING SMALLPOX FROM THE GLOBE

Rahima Banu, a three-year-old girl from a mud and bamboo hut in Bangladesh, was the last person on earth to suffer from the oozing pustules and pain of variola major, the most severe type of smallpox. She recovered from the disfiguring disease in October 1975.

In 1977, the last known case of variola minor, a less troublesome but still contagious type of smallpox, occurred in Somalia, on the Horn of Africa.

These two cases were the final link in a chain of death and destruction that had plagued humanity since history was first recorded. The chain was not easily broken. That accomplishment is a testament to the hard work of concerned health workers and to the miracles that can arise from drugs—in this case, a simple vaccine for smallpox. Thanks to a monumental international effort and the safe and quick manufacture of the vaccine, no one now need worry about waking up to the pustules and fever that characterize the once dread, but now dead, disease.

Dread was certainly justified, as this description from 17th-century England illustrates: "The small pox was always present, filling the churchyard with corpses, tormenting with constant fear all whom it had not yet stricken, leaving on those whose lives it spared the hideous traces of its power, turning the babe into a changeling at which the mother shuddered, and making the eyes and cheeks of the betrothed maiden objects of horror to the lover."

Scientists have confirmed that Ramses V, an Egyptian pharaoh who died in 1157 B.C., was a victim of smallpox. After viewing scars on the mummy, one scientist wrote, "I am almost as convinced that he did indeed have smallpox as if I had actually seen a 3,000-year-old pox virus."

Feared in the Old World, it accidentally became a major weapon in conquering the New. Hernando Cortez and his sea-weary band of 500 conquistadors were greatly aided in their conquest of Mexico by the smallpox virus. The Aztecs and other Indians had no resistance to the variola, thus the pox introduced by the Spaniards was at least as effective as Spanish ballistics in causing the downfall of a once-proud empire.

Though the pox was the scourge of the world for centuries, many cultures had at least slightly effective methods of controlling the ravages of the disease. People of China, Africa and India had for centuries practiced a technique scientists call variolation—blowing ground smallpox scabs into the nasal passages of healthy people in order to stimulate the body's immune system without causing a full-blown case of smallpox. In 1706, an African slave in Boston told Cotton Mather of this technique.

FARMER INFECTS FAMILY WITH POX

The beginning of the end of smallpox came in 1774 when an English farmer inoculated his wife and two sons with a variety of pox taken from the pustules of an infected cow. This disease, appropriately called cowpox, was rarely contagious among humans. Yet it was so similar to smallpox that it stimulated the body to build an immunity to that human disease, which was raging over the countryside.

Then, 22 years later, in 1796, Edward Jenner, M.D., took pus from the hands of a milkmaid who had become infected with cowpox. He then immunized an eight-year-old English country boy by putting the sample into an open wound, and thus eventually into his bloodstream. Two months later he tried to infect the boy with smallpox. The pox didn't take, and Dr. Jenner spread word of his success with vaccination. By 1801, more than 100,000 people in England had been vaccinated against the pox, and word of this technique was spreading. Dr. Jenner expressed the belief that "the annihilation of smallpox—the most dreadful scourge of the human race—must be the final result of this practice." Little did he know that almost two centuries would pass before his prediction came true.

Dr. Jenner's vaccination technique required that the virus be taken from a cowpox sore and passed to a healthy person. Transferring this small amount of the virus would cause the healthy person's immune system to defend against a possible invasion of the deadly smallpox. This method of passing the virus presented logistical problems: Without needles, measured doses and ways to store the vaccine, mass vaccination was difficult. It was not possible to vaccinate millions of people against smallpox by passing the cowpox from body to body. And it remained impossible until the mid-20th century and the advent of modern methods of making vaccine.

SUCCESS SEEMS POSSIBLE

A dried smallpox vaccine was introduced in West Africa in 1909, but it wasn't until 1949 that a freeze-dried vaccine was developed, finally clearing the route for eradication of smallpox. Several seriously infected areas, including India in 1962, established eradication programs. Finally, in 1966, the World Health Assembly accepted a goal that had been proposed by the Soviets many years

previously: They would wipe smallpox from the face of the earth. Then, to make the job easier, the bifurcated needle, which holds several doses at a time, was developed in 1968. This needle made vaccination relatively painless and fast. The age-old battle against the pox was finally changing gears. After so long, humanity began to beat the virus that had pummelled it for so long.

The task took cooperation and health detective work on a scale never before seen. At least 50 countries with a total population of over one billion needed to be cleared of the pox. First, volunteers fanned through a country—the slums, backcountry shanties and wealthy neighborhoods—vaccinating everyone who had not yet been exposed to the disease. In the end, due to logistics, only about 80 percent of the people who needed the vaccine received it, so small outbreaks continued to be reported here and there. Health workers quickly responded, even if they had to hike into the bush, vaccinating everyone who needed it. The existing cases were closely monitored so they wouldn't spread the disease further.

LAST CASE FOUND

As the number of cases decreased, it was less easy to track the disease. Rewards were offered in some countries to anyone who reported a smallpox case. In 1975, the world's last case of variola major—the deadly pox—was reported in Bangladesh. But the backcountry of Ethiopia was still infected with the minor pox. Ethiopia had almost no health-care network and few roads—most people lived more than a day's walk from a road—and was in the midst of both a famine and a civil war. Clearly, the country wasn't in an ideal position for a health crusade. Nonetheless, determined health-care providers, both on foot and in helicopters, fanned through the countryside vaccinating the unafflicted and isolating the victims. Just as the World Health Organization was ready to hail a victory over smallpox in Ethiopia, trouble hit. Nomads spread the disease across the border into Somalia.

11

No one wanted to lose the hard-fought battle against the pox, so Somalia declared a national emergency. More than 3,000 cases occurred in the country, but the smallpox was kept under control. Finally, the last case was isolated. Smallpox had been wiped from the earth. Not a single case of naturally occurring smallpox has since been discovered.

The cost of this miracle? About $300 million (one-eighth the amount NASA spent putting a man on the moon) for 2½ billion doses of vaccine administered by slightly more than 200,000 people, many of them volunteers. Eradication of smallpox will save the world an estimated $1 billion a year that would have been spent caring for victims of the disease.

USHERING IN THE AGE OF DISASTERS

At the same time the smallpox vaccine was beginning to banish a disease from the planet, another drug was quietly creating a new and horrifying health problem. Thalidomide, sold as a harmless sleeping pill and finally banned because it scarred forever the lives of thousands, is an example of the destructive fury of some pharmaceuticals.

Thalidomide also serves as a chilling reminder that drugs developed and marketed without extreme care can turn out to be much more harmful than beneficial. The lesson this medication teaches us is that everything is not as it seems. In this case, thousands of infants were deformed by a "harmless" drug.

Thalidomide was first synthesized in Switzerland in 1954. It caused no reaction—good or bad—in laboratory animals, and was set aside. Soon a West German company noticed that thalidomide's chemical structure was that of a sedative, and they experimented with using it to prevent epileptic seizures in humans. While it didn't work as intended for epileptics, it did prove to have a powerful hypnotic effect on people. Thalidomide worked quickly to give a deep, almost natural sleep with no morning "hangover."

It was soon available without a prescription throughout West Germany. It seemed safe. Even people who used high doses in suicide attempts suffered few ill effects. The drug was sold in combination with other agents as a treatment for everything from colds to asthma. A liquid form was sold that was used to calm anxious or noisy children. And, tragically, because the drug combated nausea, it was taken by pregnant women.

As the drug became widely used, some people began to associate it with side effects such as tingling hands and motor and sensory disturbances. This prompted West Germany to restrict the drug to prescription sales, but its popularity grew. Other countries, most of which sold the drug only by prescription, were reporting great success with thalidomide, and it was widely used.

STUBBORN FAMILY PROMPTS INVESTIGATION

At about this time Karl-Hermann and Linde Shulte-Hillen were prepar-

U.S. Escapes Tragedy

Thalidomide was not sold in the U.S., but this seems less a confirmation of the foresight and diligence of the U. S. Food and Drug Administration (FDA) than a simple matter of good luck. In fact, the Merrell Company asked the FDA in September 1960 to grant it permission to sell thalidomide. Even though the dangers of thalidomide were unknown, the FDA denied permission because the company hadn't filled out the correct papers. During the delay, indications that thalidomide might be harmful surfaced quietly in Europe, prompting Frances Oldham Kelsey, M.D., of the FDA, to ask the company to prove the drug's safety. This final delay saved the day. While Merrell was running tests, the tragedy of thalidomide became crystal clear when numerous deformed babies were born in West Germany. So the FDA denied approval of thalidomide, thus preventing a similar tragedy in the U.S.

ing to have their first baby. Karl was doing well as a lawyer, and the Shulte-Hillens were excited about starting their family in the Ruhr Valley of West Germany. Six weeks before their child was due, Karl's sister gave birth to a girl with tiny, deformed arms, and the doctors blamed it on heredity. Neither family had any history of birth defects, so the explanation was puzzling.

Linde Shulte-Hillen was having natural childbirth, and the delivery went easily until the baby, later named Jan, entered the world. The first sign of trouble came when the midwife asked Linde: "Is your husband armless, by any chance?" Karl was waiting outside the delivery room when the doctor appeared to tell him he had a son. When the doctor dropped his head sadly, Karl knew what the problem was: His baby, like his sister's, was deformed.

The problem: phocomelia, from the Greek words *phoke,* meaning seal, and *melos,* meaning limb. Phocomelic children are born with underdeveloped arms, perhaps one-fifth the normal length, and their hands often lack the proper number of fingers. The appendages on the young appear about as useful for human activities like tying shoes and driving a car as would be the flippers of a seal.

Phocomelia is extremely rare and usually affects only one arm. So it's surprising that the pediatricians would so easily dismiss two cases occurring in such a narrow period of time. Karl Shulte-Hillen would not accept heredity as the explanation, especially after finding that a friend had a child born with similar defects. This prompted him to look around, and he easily found 12 more examples of phocomelia in the immediate area. Still, health officials were not interested in his findings. Their lack of concern was unfortunate and also surprising. In 1960, most pediatric clinics in West Germany had encountered phocomelic infants. There were 27 in Munster, 30 in Hamburg and 19 in Bonn. In the years 1949 to 1959 there had been perhaps 15 cases in all of West Germany. By 1961, Jan's first year on earth, there were hundreds of cases all over the country.

HORRORS IN THE WHITE PILLS

Karl Shulte-Hillen finally found a doctor, Widukind Lenz, who would listen. After visiting several affected children, Dr. Lenz concluded that the cause of their deformity wasn't heredity but something in the environment. Lenz checked whether cosmetics, food, detergents or even nuclear fallout could be the cause. Each item was systematically eliminated from the list of suspects. Dr. Lenz then circulated a questionnaire among the mothers of phocomelic babies and noticed that a popular tranquilizer, Contergan, had been taken by many of them. Karl Shulte-Hillen then recalled a sad day: Linde's father had died when she was one month pregnant. Everyone was upset and Linde's sister passed out some white pills. Linde's sister took two, Karl and his brother-in-law took two, and Linde took two. Other mothers of phocomelic children also recalled taking white pills. The chemical which bound the pills—and the babies— was soon found to be thalidomide.

Dr. Lenz became convinced of the danger of thalidomide. He notified the chemical company by phone and registered mail that of 130 cases of phocomelia, Contergan was definitely involved in 117. The company did nothing.

Five days later in Dusseldorf, Dr. Lenz spoke before a meeting of West German pediatricians, almost all of whom had noticed an alarming increase in the number of deformities among newborns. Dr. Lenz said he had traced the outbreak to a new drug used as a sedative. He didn't name the drug, but after the meeting the doctors generally knew that Dr. Lenz suspected Contergan.

Six days later the chemical company withdrew thalidomide from the market. The Ministry of Health followed with a warning against Contergan that was picked up by newspapers and radio stations across the country.

Meanwhile, purely by coincidence, W. G. McBride, M.D., of New South Wales, Australia, also noticed an increased number of phocomelic babies. He traced them to a drug,

Distaval, and notified the Australian branch of the London chemical company that made it. This report and the news from West Germany caused the firm to stop selling the drug on December 3, 1961. Though sale of the drug was halted, phocomelic babies appeared over the next seven months or so, as mothers who had taken the drug early in pregnancy—it had to be taken during or near the second month of pregnancy to cause a problem—gave birth.

However, the tragedy continued long after the last drug-induced phocomelic birth. Thousands of babies who survived early problems grew up with limited use of their arms, unable to zip their pants without the aid of a string and a hook, barely able to clasp their hands in front of their chests, never able to walk down a street without anticipating awkward glances or disgusted stares.

Some good did come from the thalidomide disaster, however. Stiffer laws were passed in many countries to prevent further tragedies. The United States instituted strict and sometimes cumbersome regulations to limit the possibilities of another thalidomide generation.

THE DES CHILDREN

She's 27 and ready to take on the world. After establishing herself as a first-class television producer at a major-market station, Wanda decided to tackle a new and equally challenging profession: She's training to be a stockbroker. She's young, ambitious and attractive—the world is stretched out before her like a challenging game. Strolling across the Brooklyn Bridge on a balmy New York day, Wanda is trim and rosy, with a bounce in her step. A prime example of health, it seems. But health is one thing Wanda doesn't take for granted. She can't.

"My mother told us about taking DES a few years ago. Since then I try not to think about it a whole lot. But my brother had a benign tumor. He had to have surgery. And my cervix is misshapen. I've never tried to have children. I don't know if I ever will. I try not to think about it."

Wanda is one of what have come to be known as "DES children." Their mothers took a drug that was supposed to help them reach full term in pregnancy. Years later, they found that this "wonder drug" would cause them to live in quiet fear for their children's future.

The startling truth about DES is that doubts about its safety should have existed from the time it was synthesized, and confidence in its usefulness should have been trashed by two negative studies that were conducted at the height of DES use. Yet DES was widely prescribed on into the 1970s. How did this tragedy occur?

HISTORY OF A MISTAKE

DES (diethylstilbestrol) was first synthesized in 1938 as an easy-to-administer alternative to the "female" hormone estrogen, which then could be given to humans only in the form of costly injections. DES was different chemically from estrogen, but it had similar effects on the body—one of which, it was believed at the time, was to lessen the chance of miscarriage.

And DES was known to be similar to estrogen and other hormones in one other way: It caused cancer in some test animals. According to Robert Meyers, author of *D.E.S.: The Bitter Pill*, technical journals of the time reported that the offspring of DES-treated animals had physical deformities. Still, the drug was approved by the FDA in 1941 for use in treating certain hormonal disorders. The possible reasons for approval: DES was inexpensive, it could be taken orally and it was easily manufactured. Also, there were few drug-testing regulations at the time. The fear that inhibits us in the aftermath of drugs like thalidomide and DES did not exist then.

The drug did not become widespread until the late 1940s, when it was approved for use in preventing miscarriages. The year was 1947, a baby boom year, and the miscarriage rate among American women was one in four. DES was believed to be the answer to these aborted pregnancies, and doctors passed it out like so much aspirin.

Over the next ten years millions of women were given DES to help them have babies, yet there was no real proof that it worked. In fact, studies conducted at the University of Chicago showed that DES was ineffective in preventing miscarriages. Still, physicians continued to prescribe the drug out of ignorance, disbelief or habit. Though there was no proof at the time that DES was effective, neither was there evidence to suggest that it was harmful. That didn't come until much later.

THE STORY UNFOLDS

The evidence that DES was harmful began to surface in 1966 when a Massachusetts General Hospital gynecologist noticed clear cell adenocarcinoma—a rare type of cancer that usually occurs only in women over age 50—in a 15-year-old-girl. A week later another case surfaced. By 1969, eight unusual cancer cases were noted. An investigation showed that each one was tied to exposure to DES.

This study, the first clear-cut indictment of DES, was published in April 1971. Soon other physicians found similar correlations between DES and cancer. The FDA was notified, but took no action. The reasons for the delay are unclear, but the agency did not officially announce that DES was dangerous for pregnant women until November 1971, one day before a congressional hearing on DES safety was to begin. Perhaps 20,000 American women took DES in the time between the publication of the study and the FDA action. It's possible that 20,000 additional families were left to wonder whether DES would leave its horrible legacy with them.

EQUAL-OPPORTUNITY DRUG

A climate of fear was established among DES daughters in the early 1970s, but many DES mothers were able to breathe a sigh of relief and say, "Thank God I had a son."

The collective sigh did not last long. It became clear in the early 1980s that DES sons had a higher-

A DES Son Tells His Story

Craig Diamond grew up in L.A. and always pictured himself moving out of the city to the mountains when he was about 40 years old.

At 26, he was a rising young lawyer with a big Los Angeles firm representing companies being sued for selling DES.

Because Diamond felt occasional chest pains—breast pain, really—and was losing weight that first year with the law firm, he went to see a physician. "Take 2 aspirin and don't worry about it," said the doctor. So Diamond continued to work hard, sometimes visiting 3 courthouses in a single day to help with the DES lawsuits.

Finally, in early November 1980, Diamond encountered a bottle of cheap gin that saved his life. He drank too much and the hangover continued all day Sunday, all day Monday and on into Tuesday afternoon. Prompted by a friendly co-worker, Diamond took some "hair of the dog"—a shot of bourbon—to quell his ache. An hour later he noticed his urine was as dark as the bourbon. "Some friends suggested it might be a bleeding ulcer," says Diamond, who made an appointment with a doctor. "When I casually mentioned the breast pains I had been feeling," he says, "the doctor became alarmed."

Seven days later a biopsy revealed 4 different types of cancer in Diamond's right testicle. The testicle was removed, but the pain had just begun. A few days later Diamond was "split like an orange" so the surgeon could remove as many lymph nodes from his pelvic area as he could find. The resulting suffering caused Diamond to reevaluate his concept of pain. Everything else now pales in comparison.

Diamond left the L.A. law firm to live and work in Grass Valley, a small California mountain town. Having learned that his mother had taken DES and that his cancer was possibly the result, he's suing "many different companies," as well as the first physician he visited—the one who told him to take aspirin for his breast pains.

Whatever the outcome of the court cases, says Diamond, "I can honestly say that all the money in the world wouldn't make up for my losses. I live with cancer. I am disappointed with the people who are responsible for my damages. I always thought that when I was 40 I would have a long time to live in the mountains. Then I got cancer when I was 26, and 40 looked a long time away."

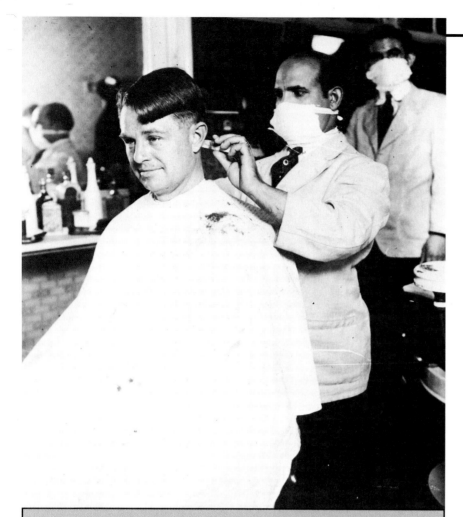

1918 Epidemic Remembered

Gussie Gaskill, now retired from her job as curator of 2 special collections at Cornell University's library, remembers the great flu epidemic of 1918, when she was 20: "I was asked to help care for some of the more serious cases among a group of soldier boys who had been sent to study at the University of Kansas, in Lawrence. About a thousand of them had come. They registered for school, got their barracks assignments, went to a few classes and came down with the flu—just about that fast. The university was closed for about 5 weeks or so.

"Everyone wore cotton or gauze masks around town to protect them from the germs. I never caught the flu, probably due to my strong constitution. People were scared, because so many people died from the flu, but no one got too depressed. That is because Kansans are little disturbed by difficulties, what with too much rain, too little rain, dust storms, cyclones and other problems. You just made it through. Still, we were glad when it ended."

than-normal chance of suffering genital abnormalities such as undescended testicles, undersized penises and ineffective sperm. Testicular cancer is believed by some to also be a side effect of DES, because there is a direct correlation between undescended testicles and cancer.

Despite the growing list of dangers, DES was never banned for use by pregnant women. The FDA only *suggested* that it not be used. According to Casey Morrigan, coordinator of DES Action in San Francisco, there have been instances since 1971 when DES was given to pregnant women. "You wonder how anyone could be ignorant of the danger associated with DES," exclaims Ms. Morrigan, "but some doctors apparently are."

DES is now commonly used to treat a number of disorders, including prostate cancer, and in estrogen replacement therapy for postmenopausal women, although no one knows the long-term effects of the drug. "What will happen to DES daughters when they get older?" asks Ms. Morrigan. "All women over 50 are already at a higher risk for cancer, including those types resulting from natural hormonal changes. Estrogens are known carcinogens." The questions Ms. Morrigan raises are: Will DES daughters suffer further? Is it safe to use DES for estrogen replacement therapy in older women?

"DES is a disaster," Casey Morrigan states flatly. She speaks from experience: She is a DES daughter. "DES has a profound effect on people's lives, even if they don't get cancer. At first you can be preoccupied with it, powerless. Then you have to educate yourself. With knowledge you become powerful, because then you learn what medical steps to take. But DES is a disaster."

THE RISE AND FALL OF ORAFLEX

The more than 30 million Americans who suffer the frequently searing and unforgiving pain of arthritis have leapt at many cures for their disease. And they always have been disappointed, because even the very best medicines only worked to control the pain and other symptoms of arthritis. None worked on the disease itself.

Suddenly, hope was bright on the horizon. A new drug, Oraflex, seemed to actually slow arthritis. It promised to be the first arthritis drug to do more than simply treat symptoms.

It was first released in England, and then two years later in the United States. It arrived with a publicity blitz that hailed it as a safe alternative to the only other effective drug relief, high doses of aspirin or aspirinlike drugs that often irritated the stomach lining. In addition, not only did Oraflex relieve arthritis pain and slow the disease itself, it also came in convenient, once-a-day doses. This aspect of the drug was seen as a big benefit for those used to running to the medicine cabinet throughout the day — and night. It seemed like a great boon for humanity, for a short time at least.

As the drug became used with some frequency, side effects were noticed. The most serious of these was damage to the liver — damage so severe that death resulted.

Within three months of this most promising drug's release in the United States, it was pulled from the market in both the U.S. and England.

THE SWINE FLU SNAFU

The flu usually isn't considered a very dangerous ailment, just a miserable nuisance. But, in truth, 17,000 people die each year from influenza and resulting complications. And when an epidemic rages, the death toll can be higher than that of a war: 65,000 in 1958; 68,000 in 1968; 500,000 in the 1918 swine flu epidemic.

Given these figures — especially the last one — it's not surprising that federal health officials were alarmed by the suggestion that swine flu was about to ravage the country again in 1977. But their response — wholesale vaccination of the population, resulting in a number of deaths and injuries — was a bit extreme, given the facts.

First, flu epidemics occur in ten-year cycles. The next wasn't due until 1978. Second, when a soldier at Fort Dix, New Jersey, was said to have "died of swine flu," triggering vaccination panic, he actually died because he aggravated his illness with a 5-mile march. It is "doubtful that he would have died had he remained in his quarters," according to Dr. Albert B. Sabin, inventor of the live polio vaccine and an adviser to President Gerald Ford on the swine flu problem. Third, according to Dr. Sabin, the vaccination panic was fueled by fear that the anticipated epidemic would be as severe as that of 1918, even though no clear connection between the two could be made. In fact, the virus that caused the 1918 epidemic had never been isolated.

Still, U.S. health officials urged President Ford to play it safe and vaccinate every man, woman and child in America. Congress responded positively to the president's appeal for $135 million to manufacture and distribute the vaccine. The vaccination juggernaut began to roll and continued until 40 million people were inoculated, even in the face of these events:

- The virus didn't evolve into the expected epidemic. It failed to spread anywhere in the U.S. or in the world.
- The four drug companies that hurriedly produced millions of doses of vaccine didn't do a very good job. In fact, only one type of vaccine produced an "acceptable response" in those aged 25 or under.
- The drug companies refused to make the vaccine unless the U.S. government assumed liability for all possible lawsuits associated with the program.

The result of this poorly administered, expensive vaccination program? Not too many died of the flu, but it is doubtful that the vaccine had anything to do with it. In fact, the vaccine itself caused a few deaths. Some 532 people developed Guillain-Barré syndrome, an ill-defined disease that causes paralysis, allegedly as a result of the flu vaccine. Twenty-three of them died. On December 16, the vaccination program was suspended. It was, according to Dr. Sabin, "poor health practice."

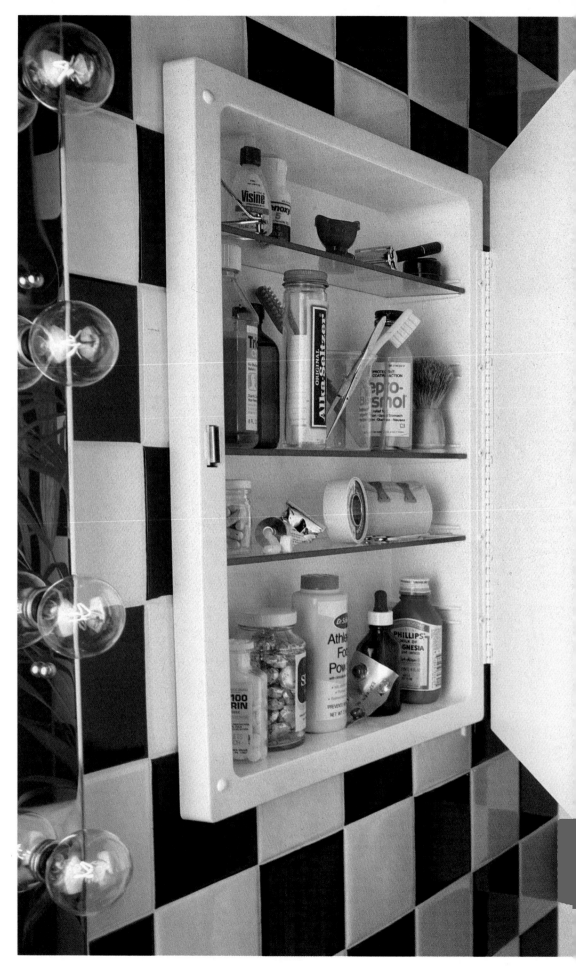

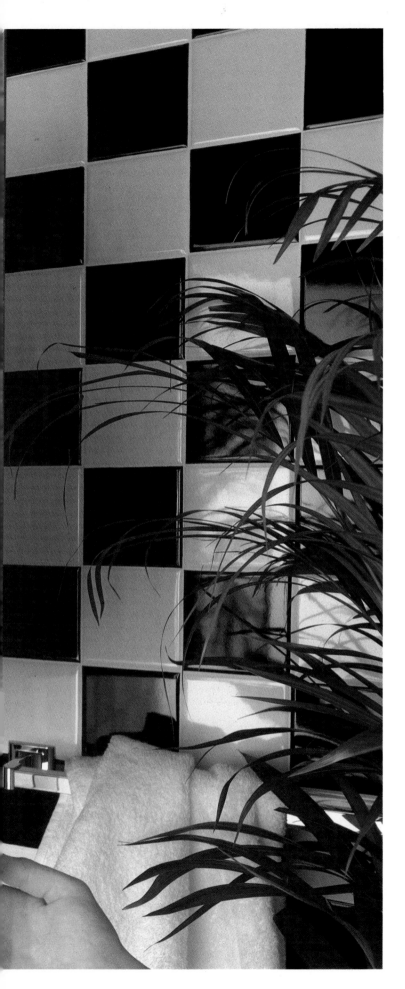

2

Everyman's Medicine Chest

We take them for granted, these over-the-counter drugs. But we shouldn't, because they're good self-help tools.

How do you spell relief? OTC, that's how. These letters stand for over-the-counter and represent all those medications we can buy without a prescription. Generally—inexpensively and very conveniently—we can dry up a runny nose, cancel a cough, take the ouch out of sunburn and the itch out of athlete's foot. Usually this sort of self-treatment involves little more than a trip to the corner drugstore or supermarket. Grouped according to their function, over-the-counter drugs can easily be scanned for range of price or dosage.

It's wonderful to have these drugs available to us. And it's wonderful to save the money that might have been spent on a doctor's bill. What's not wonderful is that these drugs are in such easy reach—so brightly packaged, sold in the aisle next to the corn flakes—that we often don't take them seriously. We just take them, often without giving them a thought.

Even though they don't require a prescription, OTC medications are *real* drugs. Like prescription drugs, some should not be combined with others or with certain foods or alcohol. Like other drugs, some can mask more serious problems or cause dependency. And sometimes an OTC drug simply should not substitute for a visit to the doctor.

Nevertheless, most are safe and effective, just as the advertisements claim. They do the job and do it well. Potential problems, however, can come from misuse or abuse. For that reason, if you're going to stock these self-help tools in your medicine chest, you'd be wise to do what you'd do with any other tools: Learn to use them wisely and learn what precautions they may require.

Acne Treatments

Truth in Advertising

The ads were so wholesome. Pat Boone and his daughter Debbie, in the service of Acne-Statin, claimed this drug a "scientifically proven" acne fighter.

Not so, said the Federal Trade Commission (FTC). They filed suit and had Boone promise to pay a portion of any court settlement.

As the FTC later explained, we often forget OTC products are *drugs*. When we buy them, we're acting as our own doctors. So we "must have access to accurate information . . . to make . . . an intelligent decision about whether to take the drug." In other words, ads can't lie.

Scrubbing your face won't get rid of it. Increasing, decreasing or halting sexual activity won't get rid of it. Even courageously declining chocolate mousse won't get rid of it. Acne isn't caused by dirt, sex or diet and won't respond to changes in them. It is caused by a genetic quirk; for some reason, in people who are acne-prone, the excess skin oil (sebum), produced at puberty, mixes with bacteria and cells living at the base of hair follicles. This creates a plug, blocking the pore and leading to a "pimple." No bacterial soap, liquid cleanser or scrub pad can have any effect on acne, because it is not caused by surface oils, nor can any of these products "plunge deep," as some advertisers claim.

If you have acne, though—as at least 85 percent of all teenagers and 20 percent of all adults in this country do—you've probably tried some of these products, lured by their claims of acne "cures." Ignore them. "No known cure is available at this time," according to Irwin I. Lubowe, M.D., professor emeritus of dermatology at New York Medical College. But, with well-considered, conscientious applications of certain drugs, acne can be controlled.

BANISH THAT BLEMISH

The U.S. Food and Drug Administration has judged only three non-prescription drugs "safe and effective" in the treatment of acne: sulfur; the combination sulfur/resorcinol; and benzoyl peroxide. Of these, benzoyl peroxide is currently acknowledged to be the most effective.

But sulfur was, until recently, the ingredient found in virtually all brand-name acne fighters. (Clearasil Acne Treatment, for example, was originally a sulfur/resorcinol product. It now contains benzoyl peroxide.) Sulfur, alone or in combination with resorcinol (they are both astringents), acts on the "peeling principle."

According to this once-popular theory, drying your face severely enough so that surface skin peels off should loosen the follicle plugs and prevent them from becoming full-blown pimples. We now know this simply isn't so; the plug is seated too deeply. Sulfur and sulfur/resorcinol products *cannot* prevent pimples.

Sulfur *can* help to dry out existing pimples. The blemishes then heal in less time than they would require if left untreated. Also, sulfur may be incorporated into flesh-colored creams, which can camouflage blemishes. So sulfur can be useful in clearing and covering the pimples you already have; it can't stop new ones.

ONE CAN PREVENT ACNE

The only over-the-counter drug that can *prevent* acne is benzoyl peroxide, available now in many brand-name products. "Benzoyl peroxide is not necessarily the silver bullet; it is just the best available treatment for acne today," says James E. Fulton, Jr., M.D., Ph.D.

As the name implies, it's a kind of bleach, which has the ability to make your skin peel plus the ability to bubble down into your pores, loosening impactions and killing the bacteria that cause pimples.

Unfortunately, many pharmaceutical companies have been adept at making their benzoyl peroxide ineffective. They set it within a base loaded with acne-causing ingredients such as isopropyl myristate. (See "The Makeup of Acne Makeup" for other villains.) Always read the labels.

A water-based gel generally works much better than a cream or a lotion, Dr. Fulton says. Too many drug companies have been operating under the misguided conception that people won't use their product if it isn't in lotion form. Benzoyl peroxide has a strong drying action. Nobody wants dry skin, they reason, so they add lotions, which, in turn, cancel out the benzoyl peroxide's power and *increase* acne. Avoid these.

Also be wary of the instructions that accompany your medication. Most of them tell you to dab it onto existing blemishes. "Dabbing is okay as a temporary measure, but using the medication over a widespread area on your face is a very good idea," says Bernett Johnson, M.D., of the University of Pennsylvania department of dermatology.

Only spreading the medicine across the entire area where pimples are likely to develop can prevent future pimples, Dr. Fulton explains. Be careful to avoid the area around your eyes, though.

The instructions may also tell you to discontinue use if redness or irritation develops. But to be effective, the drug must produce *some* irritation —that is, consistent flaking and peeling.

"Building up slowly is the name of the game," Dr. Fulton explains. Slow buildup helps prevent overdrying.

Start your treatment with a low level of exposure. Wear the medication for only 2 to 3 hours. As the skin adjusts, slowly lengthen the amount of time you wear it. The idea is to maintain consistent flaking.

TIPS TO HELP THE DRUG

To hasten recovery, wash your face before applying the drug. But don't scrub! "Soap does not help acne," says John R. T. Reeves, M.D., a dermatologist in San Francisco, "and acne medications are much more likely to sting if used on a face that has been vigorously scrubbed with soap."

After gently washing your face, chill it. Smoothing an ice cube over the skin increases benzoyl peroxide's penetration, explains Dr. Fulton. It also has an anti-inflammatory effect.

Benzoyl peroxide, used conscientiously in this way, should produce significant improvement on most types of acne within 8 to 12 weeks. But a cleared complexion doesn't mean you can quit your therapy. You must continue to use the drug until you outgrow the problem, which may take years (for men, it is usually when they're in their early twenties; for women it may be when they're in their twenties or even thirties).

Anyone with acne would agree

The Makeup of Acne Makeup

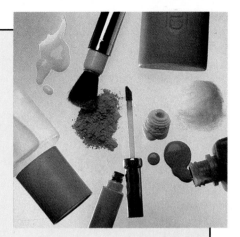

Acne is appalling enough for teenagers. Still, they usually expect it, even if they can't accept it. But today, acne in women well past their teens is blossoming out in epidemic proportions. At least 30 million women currently suffer "break-outs," caused by their cosmetics, that account for an ever-growing percentage of any dermatologist's practice. But if you suddenly sport blemishes, James E. Fulton, Jr., M.D., Ph.D., suggests you *not* run immediately to your doctor. First, try a quick and easy home remedy: Throw out all your cosmetics. "Some cosmetics ingredients are so potent that they can induce . . . acne even in women who are not otherwise acne-prone," he writes in *Dr. Fulton's Step-by-Step Program for Clearing Acne*.

Having thrown away your old cosmetics (and moisturizers, cleansers, etc.), take this list with you to your cosmetics counter and check the label on all products before you buy.

Avoid All Products with These Ingredients: Lanolins, isopropyl myristate, butyl stearate, myristyl myristate, octyl palmitate and any D and C pigments.

Look for Good Cosmetics: Almay Fresh Look Oil-Free Makeup, Bio-Clear by Med Tech, Natural Wonder Fresh-All-Day Oil-Blotting Makeup and Vaseline Dermatology Formula Cream are some examples of "safe" cosmetics. Use even these products sparingly. Remember, a clear complexion is the loveliest "look" of all.

that a commitment to treatment, no matter how prolonged, is worth it. As Dr. Fulton says, "Acne is devastating." He knows: No one could help him in his own long struggle with it. But today, though acne remains "a complicated, mysterious and devious disease, control is finally possible," says Dr. Fulton. "That is . . . joy."

Antacids

Ways to Prevent Indigestion

Yes, antacids will neutralize stomach acid. But avoiding indigestion in the first place is both healthier and cheaper. Begin by cutting out caffeine, which stimulates acid production. Avoid acidic foods such as citrus fruits and tomatoes. Also cut down on highly spiced dishes, as well as foods or substances that lower esophageal sphincter pressure, like chocolate, alcohol and tobacco.

Trim fatty foods and big meals from your life; they prolong digestion. Do wait 3 hours before going to bed even after lean, light meals, though, and try elevating your head in bed to improve stomach emptying. You'll sleep better just knowing that all of this may help spell permanent R-E-L-I-E-F.

Antacids work. Their ads may have corrupted an entire generation's ability to spell (over half the students in one nationally publicized spelling test wrote "Rolaids" when assigned the word "relief"). But, properly used, they will fight "heartburn," "sour stomach," "acid indigestion" or however *you* spell distress. Improperly used, though, they can have unfortunate, even severe, side effects.

Antacids work by neutralizing stomach acid, which is secreted abundantly to break down the food we eat. Unfortunately, the acid sometimes moves out of the stomach, where the lining is tough enough to withstand it, and migrates into the esophagus. Normally, a special muscle, or sphincter, between the stomach and esophagus prevents the acid from migrating. But at times this sphincter relaxes, allowing acid to enter the esophagus. There it irritates the sensitive lining, producing heartburn.

"Everyone gets heartburn at one time or another," acknowledges David Drake, M.D., a gastroenterologist in Long Beach, California. "When this—on occasion—occurs, almost everyone will benefit from taking an antacid of one kind or another."

But what kind? Antacids come in a whole range of different formulations, prices and even flavors. What should you look for? "It depends on your preferences and on your physical condition, on whether you have high blood pressure, bowel problems or some other health problem," says Dr. Drake. Almost all antacids today are composed of one or more of four different "active" ingredients, each with its own distinct advantages and disadvantages.

BEST INGREDIENTS

The first of these, sodium bicarbonate (Alka-Seltzer, Bromo Seltzer), has probably been quenching heartburn the longest. Also known as good, old baking soda, it's the "cheapest antacid around," says Dr. Drake. It's effective and fast acting, but it is "appropriate only for occasional indigestion," according to Gary A. Holt, R.Ph., a professor at the College of Pharmacy, University of Oklahoma, Oklahoma City.

"It is not recommended for frequent, regular use because of its high sodium content," he says. "A two-tablet dose of Alka-Seltzer [pain reliever and antacid] contains 1,102 milligrams of sodium—enough to push the dietary limits for anyone . . . who must restrict daily sodium intake," Dr. Holt explains. "If taken daily for more than a few weeks, sodium bicarbonate antacids may disrupt the acid-base balance in people with kidney problems, and contribute to recurrent urinary tract infections in women."

While original Alka-Seltzer is a pain reliever that's good for fighting a hangover or a headache, the aspirin in it can cause stomach bleeding. Look for Alka-Seltzer's Special Antacid Formula instead. It contains no aspirin.

MAJOR HELPER

Calcium carbonate (Tums, Chooz, Alka-2) is another major ingredient in antacids. It, too, is an excellent acid neutralizer, but, like sodium bicarbonate, it shouldn't be used daily for an extended period of time. Excessive intake "can raise the calcium level in the blood and may lead to impaired kidney function and possibly the formation of kidney stones," Dr. Holt says. This threat is small, though, as long as you have healthy kidneys. Some physicians even recommend Tums to help prevent osteoporosis (bone thinning).

Calcium carbonate can have other, less serious but still annoying, side effects. Prolonged use can cause constipation. It also may produce a phenomenon called "acid rebound," says Dr. Drake. This occurs when acid is produced several hours after a dose of calcium antacid, setting up a vicious cycle of acid, antacid, acid. At reasonable doses, though, calcium carbonate offers safe and effective relief.

Antigas Antacids: Bursting the Bubble

It sounds almost whimsical. "The gas that bothers you is usually 'trapped' in small, foamy bubbles," reads the label for Mylicon-80 (with simethicone.) But, thank heavens, "Mylicon-80 helps to burst these gas bubbles" so that "as the gas goes . . . so does the gas pain." And we all live unbloated ever after.

Is this just a fairy tale? Well, the facts are a little grim: The U.S. Food and Drug Administration originally declared simethicone "safe and effective," which would mean it does reduce gas. But a more recent FDA panel decided that even *if* simethicone releases bubbles (and they aren't convinced),

there's no evidence that these bubbles are actually the cause of the bloating and fullness. This opinion is echoed by the *Medical Letter*, whose consultants "found the evidence for its effectiveness unconvincing."

Should you bother, then, to pay extra money for an antacid containing simethicone? "The clinical data is scanty," admits Nicola Giacona, Pharm.D., supervisor of the Drug Information Center at the University of Utah in Salt Lake City. But, "there are some patients who swear by it. So, if it works for you, then use it."

So does magnesium hydroxide (Phillips' Milk of Magnesia). Unfortunately, it has one almost inevitable side effect: diarrhea. Most people, in fact, think of it as a laxative, not as an antacid. For this reason, it's usually found in combination with products such as aluminum hydroxide, which tend to be constipating (Gelusil, Maalox, Mylanta). If you have bowel irregularities, you might be better off using one of these.

RARELY USED ALONE

By itself, aluminum hydroxide is the weakest of the acid neutralizers. But it is not usually the sole active ingredient. Rather, it's combined with either magnesium or sodium carbonate (Rolaids). These combinations help combat constipation, but they can't totally counteract *any* aluminum-containing products' most serious potential side effect: demineralization.

Research has shown that aluminum can bind with dietary phospho-

rus and calcium, pulling them out of the body and possibly weakening the bones. In one study, volunteers given at least 2 tablespoons of antacid three times a day showed a significant increase in the amounts of calcium and phosphorus in their urine. "The calcium loss . . . may eventually result in skeletal demineralization," says Herta Spencer, M.D., one of the authors of the study. It also may cause adult rickets as well as osteoporosis.

But Dr. Spencer's study showed that an intake of at least 800 milligrams of calcium per day can help balance the effects of aluminum antacids.

If the symptoms that prompted you to take antacids in the first place persist for more than two weeks or so, see your doctor. Remember also that antacids can reduce the absorption of many drugs, including tetracycline. "Antacids aren't candy," says Dr. Drake. But, used intelligently, they are an excellent way to keep upset stomachs from upsetting you.

Aspirin and Its Alternatives

Let's try a simple word-association test. What do you think of when you hear the words "miracle worker"? Something gentle? Wearing white? In a habit? Now change the final phrase to "*is a habit*" and you've described perhaps the most remarkable miracle worker in all of medicine: the over-the-counter painkiller.

Whether aspirin or acetaminophen products, such as Tylenol, these gentle, white pills relieve pain, fever and swelling for millions of Americans. As a nation, we spend $1.3 billion a year on these products, *daily* swallowing 20 tons of aspirin alone. Why do we take so many of these pills? It's simple: because they work.

"Both aspirin and acetaminophen do a great job of relieving pain and reducing fever," says Gary C. Cupit, Pharm.D., clinical associate professor of pharmacy at the Philadelphia College of Pharmacy and Science. "Just a regular dose of aspirin (650 milligrams, or two tablets) or a similar dose of acetaminophen has been shown over and over again in clinical tests to effectively reduce pain and fever."

HOW DO THE DRUGS WORK?

Not until recently, though, have tests begun to show why these analgesics are effective. In the early 1970s scientists discovered that aspirin seems to interfere with the production of substances in the body called prostaglandins. These prostaglandins are various unsaturated fatty acids which are involved in pain. They also play a role in the regulation of body temperature, contribute to swelling after an injury and are involved in the workings of both blood vessels and kidneys.

While both aspirin and acetaminophen relieve pain well, each drug works differently. Doctors are still uncertain of exactly how, but aspirin subdues prostaglandins "within the injured tissue itself," says Anthony Temple, M.D., medical director of pediatrics at McNeil Consumer Products Company. Aceta-

minophen, on the other hand, "seems to work on prostaglandins within the brain and central nervous system, where pain is perceived," he says. Acetaminophen elevates our pain threshold.

ASPIRIN IS BETTER AGAINST INFLAMMATION

Because aspirin goes to work right where the hurt is, it is more effective than acetaminophen for reducing certain kinds of inflammation. Therefore, aspirin is the drug doctors recommend if you have rheumatoid arthritis, an inflammatory disease. "In full dosage, aspirin undoubtedly has greater analgesic activity than [acetaminophen] in inflammatory conditions such as rheumatoid arthritis," says an article in the British medical journal *Lancet.*

If you have rheumatoid arthritis, though, you should be treating yourself with aspirin *only* if you're under a doctor's care. Typically, a person with moderately severe rheumatoid arthritis will take 8 to 12 aspirins a day to help fight inflammation. Taken in these dosages over a period of time, aspirin can produce undesirable side effects, often in the form of gastrointestinal problems.

"Between 2 and 6 percent of patients [taking aspirin] will have dyspepsia [stomach discomfort], nausea and vomiting, while the loss of blood in the stools may be 10 to 20 times greater than normal, depending on the dose," doctors reported in the *British Medical Journal.*

Dose and duration are the keys here. Only people "who take aspirin regularly (on four or more days a week) or in large doses (more than 15 tablets a week) are likely to suffer acute gastrointestinal bleeding or gastric ulceration," the article concludes.

"The rate is much lower for occasional use," adds Dr. Cupit. "Less than 1 percent, in fact."

Aspirin's side effects are not limited to stomach distress. It can leave its mark on you in other ways, as well. Even one tablet can prevent platelets (tiny cells that help the blood to clot) from clumping together to form blood clots. A dose of two regular-strength tablets approximately doubles the time it takes for bleeding to stop. Moreover, this condition can last for a period of up to a week, reports an article in *Pharmacy International*. Because of this effect, check with a physician before taking any aspirin prior to surgery. It's known that it can increase postoperative blood loss.

AVOID ASPIRIN DURING PREGNANCY

A woman "in her third trimester should not take aspirin under any circumstances," emphasizes Carol Rumack, M.D., associate professor of radiology and pediatrics at the University of Colorado Health Sciences Center.

Taking aspirin regularly during pregnancy can delay and prolong labor and increase the risk of anemia, hemorrhage and other complications. Dr. Rumack explains that her research has shown that aspirin taken by the mother may increase a premature infant's chances of developing a dangerous brain hemorrhage.

"We can't prove absolutely that the aspirin was at fault," she says. But the best way to avoid possible birth complications is to avoid aspirin. "It takes a week for your body to replace the platelets affected by aspirin. During that entire week, your blood will not coagulate normally. The problem is that no one ever expects to deliver prematurely. They think things are going along just fine"—until they suddenly go into labor. If you're pregnant, "ideally you should take no drugs. But if you do want a mild painkiller," Dr. Rumack says, "make sure it's acetaminophen."

ASPIRIN IS NOT KID STUFF

Acetaminophen is also the best choice when you're deciding what to give a sick child. "Young children are particularly susceptible to the toxicity of [aspirin], and the overzealous and misguided administration of aspirin by parents (and even doctors), often for trivial complaints, may end in tragedy," the *Lancet* article reports.

Aspirin is especially dangerous when your child has a viral infection, such as chicken pox or influenza, and a fever. While aspirin can reduce fever, it also may cause your child to develop Reye's syndrome (RS). Normally, RS, a nervous system disease in which the brain swells and which is sometimes fatal, is rare.

Unfortunately, it's less rare among sick children given aspirin. One study of children with RS found that 97 percent of them had taken aspirin prior to developing symptoms. Children in a second group who did not develop the disease had been given acetaminophen—also effective in cooling fevers. There "is much to be said for restricting [aspirin] use in favor of [acetaminophen], particularly in children," the *Lancet* article concludes.

The American Academy of Pediatrics (AAP) has issued its own warning. Because another recent study showed a strong link between the use of aspirin and the development of Reye's syndrome, the academy recommends that children with the flu or chicken pox *not* be given aspirin.

SAFE UNLESS ABUSED

Is acetaminophen risk free? So it seems, according to the *Lancet* report: "Serious adverse reactions to [acetaminophen] taken in recommended doses are extremely rare, and used properly it must be one of the safest of all drugs."

The only serious potential danger in taking acetaminophen seems to be liver damage, and then only as a result of overdosing. In England, where acetaminophen outsells aspirin, people have died of liver failure after taking large doses of the drug. *Very large doses.* Typically, "about 15 grams [at least 45 regular-strength tablets] is required to produce serious intoxication in an adult," reports Scott E. Walker, pharmacist at a

Toronto medical center. Liver damage will probably occur in up to 70 percent of the people who take such an overdose.

It also might be wise to not mix alcohol with acetaminophen. In a study of laboratory animals at the Minneapolis Veterans' Hospital, doctors found that acetaminophen was lethal at a much lower dose for mice drinking alcohol than for mice who were teetotalers.

Still, for most of us, acetaminophen is safe. "If therapeutic doses of [acetaminophen] can cause liver damage, this must be a very rare event," the *Lancet* article says.

UNEXPECTED POWERS

Should we always choose acetaminophen over aspirin? While it doesn't reduce inflammation as well, it seems able to do everything else aspirin can, with smaller risks. Yet the answer is no—because aspirin has certain *beneficial* side effects that acetaminophen can't match. Using aspirin, for example, may reduce your risk of having a heart attack or a stroke or developing cataracts.

"I recommend that all my male patients over the age of 25 take one baby aspirin or half of a regular aspirin every day," says Herschel R. Harter, M.D., clinical professor of internal medicine at Louisiana State University. "The evidence that it can help protect against heart attack is just too abundant to ignore." In one famous study, 1,266 men suffering unstable angina (chest pain that may signal an approaching heart attack) were given either aspirin or a placebo. The number of men who eventually *had* a heart attack was 51 percent lower in the group receiving aspirin.

"Aspirin can't clear up hardening of the arteries," Dr. Harter explains. But the drug's ability to inhibit blood clotting may help prevent hardening in the first place. "I know I've been taking my daily aspirin for years without any stomach upset. And without a heart attack," he says.

Or a stroke. The evidence that aspirin helps protect against strokes is almost conclusive. Studies in the United States and Europe have shown that four aspirin tablets a day greatly reduce the risk of strokes and deaths from strokes.

A BABY ASPIRIN MAY HAVE BIG BENEFITS

Even smaller doses may do the same, believes William S. Fields, M.D., professor of neurology at the University of Texas at Houston. "The original studies were done when we had little idea of how aspirin works," he says. "Now the information we have about aspirin's effect on prostaglandins and blood clotting suggests that we may have been giving more aspirin than necessary."

His estimate is that 80 to 100 milligrams a day (about one baby

---

The New Breed of Painkiller

Since the 1950s, the drug heavyweights, aspirin and acetaminophen, have had the nonprescription painkiller arena to themselves. No longer. Now the FDA allows ibuprofen—previously available only with a prescription—to be sold over the counter. So, a newcomer steps into the limelight.

Sold under such brand names as Advil and Nuprin, ibuprofen is sort of a compromise drug. According to Thomas G. Kantor, M.D., of the New York University School of Medicine, ibuprofen is like aspirin in that it "has weak but definite anti-inflammatory properties." Like acetaminophen, it works "with considerably less adverse effect on the stomach." It's proven especially effective against menstrual cramping, postpartum pain, injuries to soft tissues and even the pain of tooth extraction.

Yet it isn't free of side effects. Some doctors fear that its frequent and prolonged use may complicate high blood pressure and kidney disease. Avoid ibuprofen if you have those problems, are allergic to aspirin or are pregnant. For most of us, it is a safe and effective option as we search for the best way to fight minor pain.

aspirin) might have the same protective power as larger doses. "Studies are being done now to test this and I think they'll prove it's so," Dr. Fields says. "But that doesn't mean you should run out and start taking aspirin every day just to prevent stroke. With a doctor's supervision, taking an aspirin a day may be worthwhile. But see your doctor first."

The same advice applies to people likely to develop cataracts, believes Edward Cotlier, M.D., of New York Hospital-Cornell Medical Center. "We did a series of retrospective studies on arthritis patients," says Dr. Cotlier. "What we found is that people taking four or more tablets over a long period of time had a much lower incidence of cataract formation." Also, diabetics, who are especially prone to cataracts, developed them at later ages if they used aspirin. Doctors believe that aspirin somehow binds with certain proteins found in the lens of the eye. Aspirin's actions keep these proteins from forming the cloudy mass that is a cataract.

HOW TO ENSURE SAFETY

One way to lessen the chance of your feeling even mild stomach irritation is to take aspirin with a full glass of liquid. For arthritics and others who must take lots of aspirin often, the new enteric-coated tablets may be real stomach savers. They're designed to dissolve in the small intestine instead of in the stomach. (See "A Pill That Bypasses Your Belly.")

This kind of coating on your pill may make it look more like candy than ever. But remember, aspirin and acetaminophen, whatever their form, are drugs. And, as such, they must not be taken with certain other medications. Don't take oral antacids, oral anticoagulants, antidiabetic drugs, corticosteroids, heparin or gout medications with even *one* tablet of aspirin. Always tell your doctor if you are taking aspirin or acetaminophen on a regular basis when he is prescribing other medications.

A Pill That Bypasses Your Belly

"It upsets my stomach" may be one of our most common complaints against aspirin. Most of us simply can switch to acetaminophen. If you have rheumatoid arthritis, though, you can't: You need aspirin's anti-inflammatory power. If you don't want the pain in your stomach, how can you bypass this problem? By bypassing your stomach. Enteric-coated aspirin can do this.

These often colorful pills are designed to withstand stomach acid; the coating doesn't dissolve until it reaches the alkaline environment of the small intestine. Because of this, the medication takes longer to reach the bloodstream, says William Bond, Pharm.D., of the Philadelphia College of Pharmacy and Science. So coated pills aren't recommended for acute, short-term pain (such as a headache).

But, says Dr. Bond, "for people who can't tolerate aspirin and especially for people with rheumatoid arthritis (who are predisposed to anemia anyway, and need to avoid stomach bleeding), the coated pills are quite valuable."

Also, get in the habit of reading labels and talking to your pharmacist. Aspirin often shows up where you least expect it, in both prescription and over-the-counter medications (cold remedies, for example).

Finally, to ensure that these little miracles of medicine are as safe and effective as they can be, don't exceed the dosage recommended on the package—no more than 12 regular-strength tablets per day.

"Even at such a relatively high dosage, aspirin is safe for most people," says Joe Veltri, Pharm.D., director of the Poison Control Center at the University of Utah. "But if you have pain that requires this much medication and persists for more than four or five days, stop taking the aspirin and see your doctor."

For most of us most of the time, a couple of aspirin or acetaminophen will help make the occasional hard knocks and headaches of modern life a lot easier to bear.

Cough and Cold Remedies

The *cold*, hard facts are: We can't avoid colds because they can be caused by any of more than 100 different viruses. We need only breathe droplets in the air or handle contaminated objects. Worse yet, despite the best efforts of science, a cold still can't be cured, only endured. "No medicine can speed the healing of a cold or any of its symptoms," says Paul Neis, M.D., of the ear, nose and throat department of the Kansas University Medical Center. "But many of the cold remedies available over the counter can make you feel better as you're healing."

If your symptoms center in your nose—the "Cad-ya-tell-I-hab-a-code? syndrome"—a trip to your local drugstore may help you breathe easier. "Antihistamines can help dry up a dripping nose," Dr. Neis says.

Antihistamines, as you'd probably guess, work by blocking the action of histamine, the chemical substance that causes redness, swelling and itching wherever it's released.

These happen to be the classic symptoms of allergies and, in fact, antihistamines are especially useful to allergy sufferers. They may also help those of us with colds. Antihistamines may effectively combat sneezing and dry up runny noses and watery eyes.

But antihistamines are not without side effects. Though an FDA advisory panel declared the drugs in nonprescription antihistamines to be safe and effective, the agency warns consumers not to give them to children under six without checking with a doctor first.

If you take antihistamines yourself, beware of drowsiness, an almost inevitable side effect. The FDA has issued press releases to warn the public: "Taking tranquilizers or drinking heightens this effect. . . . Don't plan on doing anything that requires coordination and quick reflexes—such as driving."

DECONGESTANTS CAN MAKE BREATHING TOUGHER

You also can unstuff your nose with decongestant sprays or drops. These work by decreasing the size of blood vessels inside your nose, thus decreasing the flow of blood to swollen nasal membranes. "But just as you can't flex a muscle forever, you also can't constrict a blood vessel forever," William Alan Stuart, M.D., writes in *Nasal Maintenance*. "When the small vessels . . . can't constrict any more, a rebound relaxation occurs . . . [making] it more difficult to breathe through your nose than it was before. . . . Your drippy nose is now being caused more by nose drops" than by your allergy or cold.

This so-called rebound effect has produced hundreds of thousands of decongestant junkies across the country. Researchers at the Milwaukee County Medical Complex found that 1 percent of *all* patients seen at the hospital suffered from "rhinitis

---

Alcohol for Infants?

A recent study by the American Academy of Pediatrics strongly criticized the alcohol levels in more than 700 liquid medicines, some of them intended especially for children. Certain cough syrups, teething preparations, decongestants and other over-the-counter drugs were found to contain alcohol in concentrations of up to 68 percent.

According to the AAP report, this alcohol may cause flushing, accelerated heartbeat, nausea and vomiting. More severe symptoms include irregular heart rate, slowed breathing and convulsions. The AAP concluded that the alcohol content in children's medicine should be limited to 5 percent at most.

"Since we published the report, one major drug company has removed alcohol from its cough syrup. I think that's a good sign," says Jean Lockhart, M.D., a pediatrician with the AAP. "Right now, though, the best way to keep alcohol out of your children's drugs is to discuss the problem with your pediatrician or pharmacist. Your pharmacist, in particular, is available and knowledgeable. He or she can tell you which drugs contain little or no alcohol. Buy them."

medicamentosa"—addiction to decongestant sprays or drops.

"*Never* use nasal spray decongestants for more than three days at the very most," warns Dr. Neis.

"Decongestants aren't harmful if you just have a cold and use them for a few days," he says. "But if your symptoms last more than ten days or if you suspect you're already dependent on decongestants, see your doctor right away. Don't deny your symptoms or try to cover them up. Cold remedies of any kind are meant to help you feel a little better for a little while. They can't do even that if you abuse them."

For a sore throat caused by a simple cold, lozenges can offer relief. Most contain a local anesthetic, Dr. Neis says, "so they are more helpful than just sucking hard candy would be. If they help you for a short time, use them."

HOW BEST TO BEAT A COUGH

A constant cough may bother you (and your family and colleagues). But if it is a "productive" cough—one that brings up phlegm—avoid using cough suppressants. Coughing "serves a useful purpose in clearing the air passages. . . . [It] is a necessary evil," an article in the *British Medical Journal* states.

If, however, you're suffering from a dry, hacking cough—one that does not earn its keep by clearing the chest—a suppressant can serve a useful function.

These drugs tranquilize the part of the brain that controls the cough reflex. "It may be legitimate to suppress the cough, especially if it interferes with sleep or work," the *Harvard Medical School Health Letter* reports. "Suppressants containing codeine or dextromethorphan . . . are effective and safe when given in correct dosages. It is especially important to measure the dosage of such medicines carefully in children."

If your cough or sore throat is being irritated by postnasal drip, "take a decongestant every 4 hours," suggests Brent Q. Hafen, Ph.D.,

Don't Make Treating Your Cough an Attack on Your Teeth

How sweet it is! And how sour that news is for our teeth.

"The hidden sugar in many nonprescription products adds to an already outrageous sugar consumption level in the United States and it adds in a significant way," writes Darlene Fujii, a registered dietitian and staff associate with the American Dental Association in Chicago, in *American Pharmacy.*

Cough drops are perhaps the worst offenders. "Children, in particular, and some adults treat minor throat irritations by continuously sucking on . . . 'medicinal candy,'" warns Ms. Fujii. This "candy" causes "untold harm to their dental health." Some cough drops contain almost 70 percent sugar.

Cough syrups can be just as villainous. In one British study, children given sweet syrups, including cough syrups, over a 6-month period had significantly more cavities than their unmedicated friends. "Liquid medicines for children should be either unsweetened or sweetened with non-cariogenic (non-cavity-causing) substances," the doctors who conducted the study concluded.

Your best defense in this attack on your teeth is to find a low-sugar product. Brands that are low enough in sugar to spare your teeth include Vicks Medicated Throat Drops (all flavors), Robitussin Cough Syrup, Robitussin-CF and Vicks Formula 44D Decongestant Cough Mixture.

Always read the label on any cough medication before you buy it, Ms. Fujii suggests. Not all labels list sugar, but some do. And remember that sucrose, dextrose and corn syrup are sugar, too.

coauthor of *Medical Self-Care and Assessment.* "Don't take antihistamines, because they dry out the lining of the throat and bronchial passages."

Remember, too, the trite but true advice: rest, keep warm and drink plenty of fluids.

Foot Care Products

Our poor feet. We walk all over them. At age 35, most of us will have tromped some 45,000 miles. Not surprisingly, as many as 90 percent of us experience foot problems.

In hot pursuit of relief, we annually spend $2 billion on over-the-counter sprays, supports, pads, powders and potions. Much of this money "is wasted, because of misinformation," says Dennis F. Augustine, D.P.M., author of *Holistic Foot Care*. But if *properly* used, these products can almost guarantee you happy feet.

To learn the ins and outs of foot products, let's begin with the ins and outs of foot problems: calluses and corns. Both are made up of dead, toughened tissue, but while calluses protrude outward, corns project inward, into the foot. Despite their difference of direction, they are treated with similar products: foot pads.

One type of pad is medicated, made of a 40 percent salicylic acid plaster that will effectively dissolve the toughened tissue. Use these medicated pads cautiously. "Yes, salicylic acid dissolves the callus. But it can't distinguish between dead cells and living tissue," Dr. Augustine warns. "If you use them once or twice, you'll be okay. But if you use them more than two or three times—as you'd have to, to remove a callus—you're going to give yourself a serious chemical burn."

*Un*medicated corn and callus pads are what you want. These do a good job of keeping you on your feet, Dr. Augustine believes. They lessen the friction between the sore foot and the offending shoe. Foam rubber inserts made of Spenco, the

Keeping in Step with the Latest Foot Aids

The names of nonprescription foot aids are not poetic. There is no music in the words bunion pad, corn cushion or moleskin. But, "for a minor foot problem, products such as those Dr. Scholl's makes can give some relief," says Dennis F. Augustine, D.P.M.

Moleskin (pictured below) is actually made of cotton flannel that you buy in strips and then cut to fit the affected area. "Moleskin is a fine way to protect calluses or corns, as well as blisters," Dr. Augustine says.

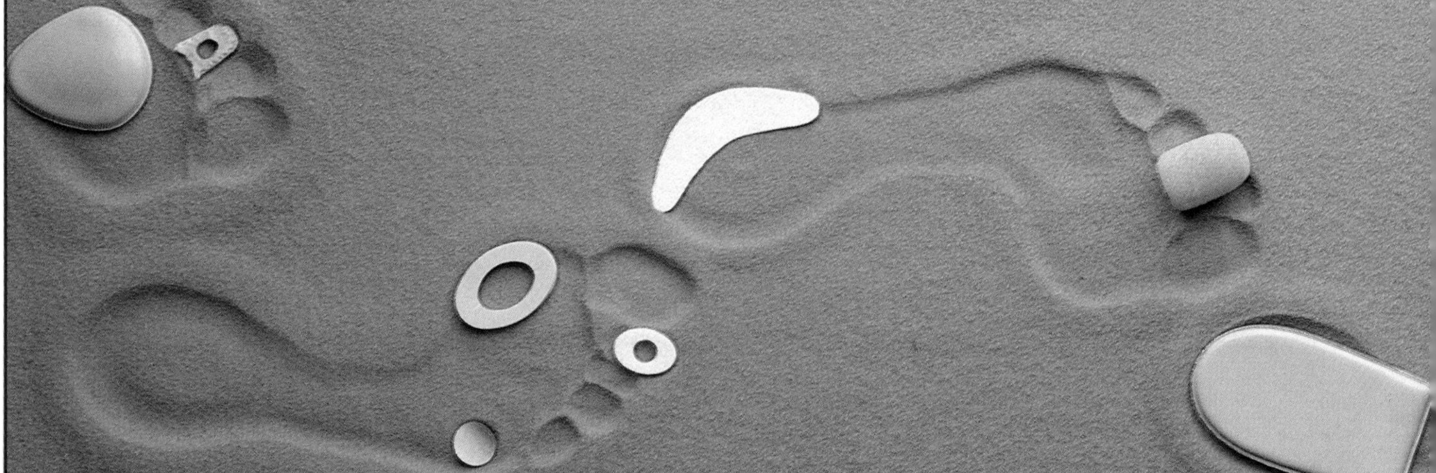

Other corn and callus products also are available and come in a variety of forms. It's important to choose the best form for a specific problem. Soft corns, for example, are those that develop between

insulated material skindiving suits are made of, are useful for calluses on your heels. Doughnut-shaped corn or callus pads are best for foot faults elsewhere; they surround the corn without putting pressure directly on the top of its painful dome.

An important footnote: Pads only make your feet feel less sore, they don't remove the corn or callus. Only softening and scrubbing can do that. Dr. Augustine suggests using a pumice stone. If you soak your feet in a vinegar bath for 20 minutes, the stone can then effectively and safely be used to file the tough skin away.

To protect this tender area, use a foam pad or moleskin (see "Keeping in Step with the Latest Foot Aids") and tincture of benzoin, an antiseptic. Benzoin has a sticky consistency that keeps the pad in place.

GIVING THE BOOT TO ATHLETE'S FOOT

Living in a shoe is tough on your foot. The warm, wet environment in there invites fungus growth, better known as athlete's foot. Luckily, nonprescription antifungals "can clear up any simple fungal problem," Dr. Augustine says.

Antifungals are available in spray, cream, liquid or powder form. "Medicated powders such as Desenex are very helpful if you perspire heavily," Dr. Augustine says.

Over-the-counter products are available to treat a whole array of other foot ills, from flat feet to soft corns. Get the correct product for your condition (in the correct size, if necessary), use it according to directions and you'll soon feel as if you're walking on air.

your toes. These require a special soft corn pad. Corns that develop elsewhere are best covered with a "doughnut-shaped cushion," Dr. Augustine says.

Products also are available for generalized foot problems. "Minor strains in your feet may be relieved with mass-produced supports," he adds. (See the metatarsal cushion, heel cushion and Ball-O-Foot cushion below.)

Foot aids such as these provide temporary relief for minor problems. Special problems may require special treatment.

"No two feet are exactly alike, any more than two eyes are," explains Elizabeth Roberts, D.P.M., professor emeritus at the New York College of Podiatric Medicine. "If you have continuing foot pain or problems, see a podiatrist."

Hemorrhoid and Diarrhea Treatments

Health problems like hemorrhoids and diarrhea embarrass us, yet they afflict most of us. At least 50 percent of all Americans develop hemorrhoids sooner or later. And almost all of us experience a yearly bout or two with diarrhea.

To find relief, we spend millions of dollars on over-the-counter remedies—which we hide under the paper towels at the checkout counter. Most of the drugs are both safe and effective, but must be used properly.

Hemorrhoids can cause discomfort or even excruciating pain. Many OTC drugs are available to help you lessen or live with this discomfort.

One type is a local anesthetic, which blocks the capacity of nerves to send information about discomfort to the brain. "If these drugs claim only to be soothing—and not to promote healing—they're at least honest," James O. Robinson, M.D., of the University of Texas Health Science Center, says.

The active ingredients in anesthetic preparations vary. An FDA advisory panel found only two to be proven safe and effective, and then only for *external* hemorrhoids: benzocaine (Lanacane and Medicone) and pramoxine hydrochloride (Tronolane).

"The use of anesthetics for a day or two is fine," Dr. Robinson says. "But overuse leads to sensitization. In effect, you become allergic to the drug. You start feeling more discomfort than before you used it. So, you use it again to get rid of the discomfort. If you have a problem that persists after a few days of using an anesthetic, see your doctor."

The same advice applies to applications of Preparation H, a popular hemorrhoid product. It's one of the remedies known as protectants; they form a protective coating on the skin, soothing itching and burning. Petroleum jelly (Vaseline), by the way, is also an effective protectant.

Some drugs claim also to shrink the swelling of hemorrhoidal tissues. Are these claims true?

"Not really," Dr. Robinson answers. "Hemorrhoids naturally pop up, then naturally disappear. If you put ointment on during the day, then they disappear, you might think the drug made the swelling go down."

However, many hemorrhoid remedies contain an astringent, which causes the skin and mucous membrane to "pucker." Though this action doesn't reduce swelling, it can provide temporary relief from itching and burning. According to the FDA, calamine, zinc oxide and witch hazel

Do You Have Hemorrhoids?

The United States spent $50 million to study the backside of the moon that never caused any of us any trouble but not one cent to study the backside of our own suffering people, says Leon Banov, Jr., M.D., a hemorrhoid specialist.

Because little information has been available, confusion and misinformation about hemorrhoids remain widespread. What *are* they? "A hemorrhoid is a gross dilation of the veins around the anal canal," explains James O. Robinson, M.D.

The inner lining of the anal canal sometimes works its way out through the anus, and the big veins in the lining become trapped. They're then stranded outside the tight muscle of the anal sphincter, which won't allow reentry.

How can you tell whether you have a hemorrhoid? The usual symptoms are pain, bleeding and/or a small, protruding lump of tissue at the anal opening. All of these may appear before or after a bowel movement, Dr. Robinson says.

"The same symptoms, though, could be caused by something more serious," he cautions. "Hemorrhoids themselves are quite treatable. But if you have any symptoms that you suspect are caused by hemorrhoids, see your doctor right away. He's the only one who can make a proper diagnosis and help you decide on the proper treatment."

are all safe and effective astringents.

In fact, witch hazel (Tucks pads and ointments) "is the best thing you can use on hemorrhoids," Dr. Robinson says.

A diet packed with fiber may also help combat hemorrhoid problems. And it's equally important if you wish to avoid another nasty gastrointestinal (GI) complaint —diarrhea. But fiber is a long-term solution. If, tomorrow, you unexpectedly find yourself making non-stop toilet stops, you'll want more immediate relief. Can over-the-counter remedies provide it?

TREATING DIARRHEA

"For someone who's healthy—not dehydrated, and only suffering from run-of-the-mill diarrhea—nonprescription products are safe and should help," says Joseph Steiner, Pharm.D., of the University of Wyoming Family Practice Residency Program.

The one ingredient in the over-the-counter drug the FDA has declared safe and effective against diarrhea is calcium polycarbophil (Mitrolan). It works by drawing water out of the body and into the small intestine, giving your stool a consistency "like oatmeal," according to Dr. Steiner. (This same action makes Mitrolan effective against diarrhea *and* constipation.)

The ingredients kaolin and pectin (Kaopectate Concentrate and Donnagel) also "pick up water like a sponge." Dr. Steiner says. "Of course, you don't want to draw water out of your body if you're already dehydrated. But dehydration normally only follows chronic diarrhea."

In the short run (no pun intended), "Kaopectate can be very beneficial. In absorbing water, it may also absorb some of the toxins that contributed to the diarrhea in the first place," says Dr. Steiner. He cautions, however, to avoid products containing paregoric, an opiate. "It does exactly the opposite of what

Can Pepto-Bismol Keep Travelers in the Pink?

"Travel expands the mind and loosens the bowels," writes Martin E. Plaut, M.D., in *The Doctor's Guide to You and Your Colon*. Every year, turista strikes 50 million of us. Fortunately, Pepto-Bismol may save the day (and the trip).

For this OTC product to be effective you must start taking it *before* diarrhea begins—even before you leave the country. In one study, students traveling to Mexico swigged 2 ounces of the pink liquid 4 times a day. They had only a 23 percent rate of diarrhea. Their untreated friends had a 61 percent rate. New research reported at the National Institutes of Health shows, however, that the optimal dose may be less: 1 ounce, 4 times a day.

For a 2-week trip, though, you'd need a lot of Pepto-Bismol. Chewable tablets are more convenient. To get the necessary coating action in your stomach, though, you have to chew the tablets for several minutes, allowing the drug to mix thoroughly with your saliva.

Also remember that, pink and innocent as Pepto-Bismol looks, it *is* a drug. It contains salicylates—one of which is a relative of aspirin. If you take enough to prevent diarrhea, you'll be swallowing the equivalent of about 8 regular-strength aspirin tablets a day. For anyone already taking large doses of aspirin—to combat arthritis, for example—that could produce dangerously high concentrations of aspirin in the blood. See your doctor before using Pepto-Bismol. Have a happy, *safe* trip.

you want: It slows down the motility (movement) of the GI tract. Because it then keeps all the toxins in place, it may, potentially, make you sicker, not better.

"Remember, diarrhea is just a symptom, not a disease." Dr. Steiner explains. "Use over-the-counter products if they make your diarrhea easier to bear—but drink plenty of fluids and eat lightly at the same time."

In sum, neither diarrhea nor hemorrhoids is anything to laugh at or blush over. Either can make you miserable, but the bother of both can be eased if you use the proper drugs properly.

Laxatives

Every year, we spend nearly $400 million on more than 700 different over-the-counter laxatives, all promising to bring relief from what is delicately called irregularity.

We call it constipation and it afflicts 41 million of us. If you're looking for relief, remember that different types of laxatives have different potential benefits and side effects.

CHEMICAL LAXATIVES

Chemical stimulants are the strongest type of laxative. Chemical names to look for are senna (Senokot, Fletcher's Castoria), phenolphthalein (Ex-Lax, Correctol, Feen-A-Mint), danthron (Dorbane), bisacodyl (Dulcolax) and castor oil.

"Stimulant laxatives are undoubtedly effective but should be used with caution, as they all produce undesirable and occasionally dangerous side effects," an article in the *British Medical Journal* warns.

Those side effects can include painful cramps, diarrhea and dehydration. But the big problem with laxatives of this type comes from abuse. Taken over a long period of time, they can become habit-forming. Addiction is bad enough, but it may be complicated by malnutrition: When taken regularly, the action of laxatives can cause a depletion of certain key minerals from the body.

Beware especially of laxatives containing phenolphthalein. When taking these, according to Jacques Thiroloix, M.D., author of *Constipation: Its Causes and Cures,* "The cells of the colon 'weep' under the assault, secreting a ropy, gluey liquid—mucus—which, mixing itself with the fecal mass, makes it more liquid." That's like bringing down a fever by locking yourself in a deep-freeze: The cure is worse than the disease.

"Of the stimulant laxatives only senna derivatives and bisacodyl can be recommended for general use, and then ideally only for short periods,"

Laxative Addiction

Are you constipated? Take this short quiz and find out: (1) Do you have 1 and only 1 bowel movement every day? (2) Do you have only 3 per week?

If you answered yes to either question, you probably are not constipated. According to W. Grant Thompson, M.D., associate professor of medicine at the University of Ottawa, "Constipation, like beauty, often 'lies in the eye of the beholder.'"

Unfortunately, some of us reach for laxatives if we go even a day without a bowel movement. The danger of using laxatives too often is that you can become dependent on them—with serious results.

Chronic use of laxatives is a little like rubbing your large intestine with sandpaper: It becomes thinner and its muscles can't work as well. "In effect, the large intestine becomes ineffective at contracting—a floppy structure," warns J. Thomas Danzi, M.D., in *Free Yourself from Digestive Pain.* You no longer can have normal bowel movements; you need a laxative just to make your large intestine work.

Is there a cure? Yes. Stop taking laxatives, states an article in the *British Medical Journal.* Of course, you may feel uncomfortable for a few days. But don't despair. And don't resort to more laxatives. Even if you've been dependent on the products for a long time, once you stop, according to the article, "bowel habit can rapidly return to normal."

the *British Medical Journal* article concludes.

WORKING BY OSMOSIS

Osmotic or saline (salt) laxatives absorb and pull water into the feces for fast relief. The most common include magnesium hydroxide (Phillips' Milk of Magnesia), magnesium sulfate (Epsom salt) and sodium sulfate.

"When taken in small doses magnesium hydroxide is useful as a laxative for simple constipation," writes Mary E. MacCara, Pharm.D., assistant professor of pharmacy, Dalhousie University, Halifax, Nova Scotia. People with kidney disease should take a different type of laxative. Writing in the *Canadian Medical Association Journal*, Dr. MacCara reports, "Up to 20 percent of the magnesium can be absorbed." She notes that high magnesium levels pose a threat to anyone with kidney problems. High levels of sodium also can be harmful to anyone with heart disease. Avoid these laxatives if you're on a salt-restricted diet.

You might try glycerin suppositories, another kind of osmotic laxative, if you occasionally need relief. They have no effect on the rest of the body and usually work within 30 minutes, Dr. MacCara explains. Rarely, they may cause rectal irritation.

MINERAL OIL

A less satisfactory laxative alternative is any of the lubricants, such as liquid paraffin or mineral oil. These act by coating the stool, allowing it easy passage.

"The use of mineral oil has many hazards and cannot be recommended," Dr. MacCara says. Taken over a period of time, mineral oil may deplete the body of all the fat-soluble vitamins (A, D, E, K). Besides, it can be messy, since it sometimes causes rectal leakage. More seriously, it can be aspirated into the lungs of elderly or bedridden patients, causing pneumonia.

Stool softeners, another type of laxative, are similar to mineral oil in that they make the stool easier to pass. But they do it less hazardously. Softeners promote the mixing of watery and fatty substances, which then penetrate the stool and soften it. The chemical involved is called DDS—dioctyl sodium sulfosuccinate.

Although DDS does not interfere with the absorption of nutrients from the intestinal tract, it has been reported to enhance the absorption of mineral oil and should never be used along with it.

Stool softeners are useful after heart or rectal surgery, when you shouldn't strain at stool, according to Dr. MacCara. But you should never use them for more than a week to ten days.

BULK LAXATIVES ARE BEST

Probably the safest of all laxatives are the bulk-forming agents, which include psyllium preparations (Metamucil, Effersyllium, Perdiem, Konsyl, Siblin) and calcium polycarbophil (Mitrolan). They work by absorbing water, then expanding. The added bulk stimulates contractions, while the absorbed water softens the stools, making them easier to pass.

Until recently, several of these products were high in sodium, but manufacturers have since cut it back considerably. Several of the preparations, however, contain as much sugar as active ingredient! Read labels carefully and choose an unflavored or low-sugar brand.

Also, make sure you drink at least 8 ounces of water or other liquid when you take any bulk-forming laxative. The liquid helps prevent blockage of the gastrointestinal tract and helps the fiber to encourage your own system to do the work.

While all laxatives do work, each type has the potential for adverse effects, particularly if used over a long period of time. Doctors say you can reduce the likelihood of problems by initiating the following practices: Get plenty of exercise, don't strain at or hurry through defecation, eat plenty of fiber and drink fluids. Doing so will help you quickly reestablish regular bowel habits without the need for laxatives.

Do Prunes Work?

Poor prunes. They're always being laughed at, when they deserve to be loved and devoured. Not only are they nutritional powerhouses, they're also one of nature's best purgatives.

The prune "is the most pleasant laxative I know," writes Edward Podolsky, M.D.

Scientists haven't yet discovered exactly *how* prunes work (their "laxative" is probably fiber), but they've proven that they do.

Nutritionists also sing the praises of prunes. While some laxatives deplete the body of vitamins, prunes *add* vitamin A and niacin and the minerals potassium, magnesium and calcium.

Oral Hygiene Products

During a lifetime of chomping, chewing, mashing, grinding and biting, our teeth take a serious beating. The result? That gap-toothed grin we find so charming in an eight-year-old may appear again, with less appeal. Just a few years ago, more than half of us could have expected to lose our teeth by the time we were 65. No more.

"Tooth loss is [not]. . .a natural consequence of aging," states an article in *Postgraduate Medicine*. Tooth problems are the result of inadequate care. Using over-the-counter oral hygiene products, you can decrease your chances of ever developing tooth or gum problems.

Smokers' Toothpaste Removes Stains—And Teeth

Ads for smokers' toothpaste are strangely reassuring. As we watch, smoke puffs through a cloth square, spreading a disgusting stain across it. The spokesman frowns. Just one cigarette can do this, he says. Imagine what an entire pack will do to. . .your lungs? No. Your teeth. They'll be stained. Smokers' toothpaste, though, removes these stains. The ad somehow implies that the harm from smoking can be undone. That—somehow—it's okay to continue smoking.

"Smokers' toothpaste doesn't seem to make much sense," comments Louis Gangarosa, M.D., professor of oral biology at the Medical College of Georgia.

"Smoking stains the teeth. Then smokers use these high-abrasion toothpastes. Dentin [the soft material beneath a tooth's enamel and on the root] can be seriously damaged by abrasives," says Dr. Gangarosa. "Unfortunately, dentin is yellow, meaning smokers may mistake it for stained teeth." They use smokers' toothpaste against these stains, and expose more, easily damaged dentin, then use more toothpaste and so on.

"But the worst thing about smokers' toothpaste," he continues, "is that it encourages people to keep smoking. If you don't want stains, I recommend you quit."

CAVITY FIGHTERS

Toothpaste can be especially useful. If teeth aren't cleaned often, plaque forms. Cavities follow. "A lot of people won't clean their teeth if they don't have minty gel on their brush," explains Allen Crawford, Jr., D.M.D., who has a family practice in Macungie, Pennsylvania. "Toothpaste is great if it gets people to brush."

But can toothpaste prevent cavities? Toothpastes containing fluoride (including Aim, Crest, Aqua-Fresh, Colgate MFP, Macleans) and carrying the "Seal of Acceptance" have the official approval of the American Dental Association (ADA). In some laboratory tests, fluoride toothpastes have been shown to reduce cavities by anywhere from 15 to 42 percent.

"Fluoride is very important when teeth are forming," emphasizes Thomas McGuire, D.D.S., author of *The Tooth Trip*. Children, however, can even get too much of a good thing. If they ingest far more fluoride than they need, their teeth become permanently discolored. This occurs rarely, but Dr. McGuire recommends you help prevent it by supervising your child's brushing. "Sometimes children think these pastes are candy and will swallow it. Teach them instead to rinse after brushing by tilting their head back and gargling. Let them learn good habits from you."

One habit you might not want to cultivate is the use of desensitizing toothpastes, which are used by people whose teeth hurt when they eat certain foods. "These have not proved to be very successful," says Norman Wood, D.D.S., Ph.D., professor of oral surgery at Loyola University.

Dr. McGuire agrees. "These toothpastes treat the symptom, but not its cause. If you have sensitive teeth, your gums have probably receded. Maybe you're brushing improperly and promoting your gum problems. A desensitizing toothpaste can sometimes block the nerve impulses and, for a day or two, that's all right. But if you don't change your habits, if you don't see a dentist, you'll wind up doing more damage," he says.

FLUORIDE MOUTHWASHES MAY WORK

Mouthwashes are not miracle workers either, but those containing fluoride can help. "Fluoride mouthwashes are very good for children, if they know better than to swallow," Dr. Crawford says. If you live in an area with unfluoridated water, Dr. Wood recommends that you rinse daily with a mouthwash containing 0.05 percent sodium fluoride, such as Fluorigard.

Don't rely on mouthwashes to mask bad breath, though. "A healthy mouth won't produce odors," Dr. McGuire says. "Infections of the gum will. If you have bad breath that lasts for more than a day, see your dentist."

Gum disease not only causes bad breath but also is the leading cause of tooth loss. Dental floss used daily helps keep your gums healthy. Some dentists recommend unwaxed floss exclusively, but if your teeth are tightly packed, it can fray, break, make you swear—or worse, make you swear off flossing.

"If this has been your experience, get some waxed floss," advises Dr. Wood. "I sometimes wonder if the dentists who so adamantly order the use of unwaxed floss really use it themselves!"

Dental tape, which is thicker than floss, may also work if you've had trouble flossing. Or try a water-spray device like WaterPik. Make sure you don't set the pressure gauge above 2½ during the first week of use, though. Gradually increase the pressure over time.

"All of these—floss, tape, WaterPik— are valuable if you use them religiously and correctly," Dr. McGuire says. "Flossing and brushing are especially complementary: what one misses, the other gets."

If, despite your careful brushing, flossing and fussing over your teeth, you still develop mouth pain, one of the self-proclaimed oral bandages (Orabase, Anbesol) may be useful

temporarily. These anesthetics contain benzocaine, which deadens the sensations of nerve endings.

"Using these products is literally like putting a Band-Aid on an open wound," says Dr. McGuire. "They're quite useful and effective in a pinch, while you're waiting to get to the dentist. But don't keep using them in place of seeing your dentist."

Dentistry has come a long way in its ability to make good dentures, Dr. McGuire says. "But if you don't wear dentures, don't let that reassure you. Don't think, 'Since they're making better dentures now, I don't have to care for my teeth.'

"Remember," he adds, "all of the readily available oral hygiene products are effective and useful if used carefully. But the final responsibility for your dental health is *yours*. You won't find the answers to your problems in a drugstore or by leaving everything up to your dentist or by blaming it on genetics. Tooth and gum problems are a little like forest fires: Only you can prevent them."

What about Disclosing Tablets?

An excellent way to keep your teeth clean and white is to dye them pink. While this suggestion sounds silly, using dye actually *is* an excellent way to keep your teeth healthy. The dye comes in the form of disclosing tablets, which stain plaque, not teeth. The chewable tablets, made of vegetable dye, are available at most drugstores or from your dentist.

"By disclosing before and after you brush, you will have a good idea of the areas you have missed and can work on these," write the authors of *Your Mouth Is Your Business*.

Use the tablets every day at first, they advise. You'll soon recognize the places in your mouth that you habitually miss and can start brushing them more carefully. "As your plaque removal improves, you should only have to spot-check once or twice a week," they say.

Be a little cautious with the tablets, though. Dye is blind: It can't tell plaque from lips, clothing or even your sink. Given the chance, it'll stain all of them. So, use a little Vaseline to protect your lips and rinse your sink thoroughly after disclosing.

Salves, Balms and Ointments

Ben-Gay before Exercising?

Exercising can make your heart, limbs and ego healthy but your muscles *sore*. Can Ben-Gay, used before a workout, prevent the aches?

Yes, reports Frank G. Shellock, Ph.D., of Cedars-Sinai Medical Center. Ben-Gay can decrease muscular discomfort, particularly in areas where you've had a muscle injury like a strain or a pull. You can then work out longer without fatigue.

Ben-Gay alone, though, can't substitute for a warm-up involving movement, Dr. Shellock says. You need to raise your heart rate and temperature before you begin. So rub in Ben-Gay, but then walk, stretch or jog slowly for a while. You'll be ensuring more fun in your run.

Not all over-the-counter drugs are made to be chewed, swallowed or injected. A large body of drugs are put on, not in, the body.

These topically applied drugs are useful in treating a variety of problems, from itching to aching. "Far too many people head to a doctor, costing themselves lots of money, for minor complaints like dandruff or poison ivy. You really should try nonprescription treatment first," suggests William Epstein, M.D., chairman of the department of dermatology, University of California, San Francisco.

TREATING THAT ITCH

One of the most common minor skin complaints is itching. Allergies, insect bites, poison ivy, dry skin—all can cause it and it can be as debilitating as severe pain, Dr. Epstein says. Though no drug can *cure* itching, many can make it more bearable.

Different kinds of over-the-counter drugs ease different kinds of itching. Hydrocortisone (Bactine Brand Hydrocortisone, Caldecort, Cortaid, Lanacort) is useful when inflammation accompanies the itching.

"The more redness, scaling, even oozing that you have, the more likely hydrocortisone is going to help. It's an anti-inflammatory drug, so it can't do much for dry noninflammatory itching," explains Paul M. Lazar, M.D., professor of clinical dermatology at Chicago's Northwestern University Medical School.

"It can be quite effective if you have eczema or poison ivy," he says. "But don't use it over your whole body. The drug can be absorbed and that may possibly lead to suppression of the pituitary-adrenal system. Be especially wary of using it where you have lots of sweat and oil glands, such as on the face, groin or underarms."

If your itching continues for more than two to three days after you start using hydrocortisone, or if your symptoms worsen, Dr. Lazar suggests that "you may have misdiagnosed your condition, or hydrocortisone just may not be the drug for you."

In this case, you might consider supplementing or even supplanting hydrocortisone with some other product. "In my own practice, I still use coal tar," Dr. Lazar says. "It works much more slowly than hydrocortisone, but it isn't as readily absorbed. When you have a large area to treat, you might use coal tar or one of its derivatives where you're the most sensitive—like the face—and hydrocortisone elsewhere." If the condition continues, Dr. Lazar advises that you see a dermatologist.

"If you itch because your skin is dry, one the best 'drugs' around is petroleum jelly (Vaseline)," Dr. Epstein says. "Other effective moisturizers are going to be available soon. Keep watching for them in your drugstore."

ANESTHETICS FIGHT ITCHING, INFECTION

Topical anesthetics also can combat itching in some people. The drugs lidocaine (Bactine First Aid Spray, Mercurochrome II, Unguentine Plus) and benzocaine (Lanacane, Dermaplast) are among the most common over-the-counter anesthetics.

"Anesthetics work great, in some cases, for some people," Dr. Epstein says. "They don't work for other people and we don't know why. If one helps you, great. Use it. But don't use it for more than a week." The reason: Overuse of anesthetics can sensitize your skin. Should that happen, you become allergic to the drug and may wind up with a worse itch than you started with. See your doctor about any itch that persists longer than a week.

Some of the anesthetics also contain antiseptics such as benzalkonium chloride, iodine or alcohol. These first-aid products claim to fight infection in minor cuts and abrasions. According to the FDA, they *cannot* claim to "promote" or "speed" healing. So, are they useful?

"They certainly can't hurt," Dr. Epstein admits. "I don't believe they can really reduce the chance of infection. But Bactine, for instance, is an effective cleansing agent."

Products containing alcohol are

also good wound cleansers, he says. "But they can be quite irritating to the skin. Wash them off quickly and thoroughly. And for heaven's sake, don't drink them."

Equally irritating and undrinkable is the once-popular antiseptic mercury, which was found in Mercurochrome. Used on a wound, it would sting and stain everything—skin and clothing—red. You won't find it in Mercurochrome any longer. You won't find it in anything else, either. An FDA advisory panel judged it safe but ineffective. Mercurochrome now contains benzalkonium chloride and alcohol for wound cleansing.

Iodine, though, which also can sting and stain, is still available. It is also "among the most potent antiseptics available," according to the *Medical Letter.* But it should be used with caution. (See "Whatever Happened to Iodine?")

Remember, clean wounds heal themselves, Dr. Lazar says. If the wound is large or ragged, see a doctor before trying self-treatment. And if it remains pus filled, swollen or painful for more than a few days or if it worsens, don't rely on antiseptics to "cure" it. Again, see your doctor.

For more widespread aches and pains, a product that's spread widely may help. Thus, if you have muscle aches, products containing methyl salicylate (Ben-Gay, Icy Hot Balm or Ointment, Mentholatum Deep Heating Rub, Deep-Down Pain Relief Rub) may be useful.

"All of these produce a feeling of warmth, which is nice," Dr. Epstein says. "Plus, the rubbing action as you put them on may act like a minimassage, loosening tight muscles. But they certainly can't penetrate to the muscle itself."

SELF-CARE IS SMART CARE

"My strongest recommendation concerning skin problems is that you don't ignore them; don't let them get to the point where you *have* to see a doctor," Dr. Epstein urges. "So

Whatever Happened to Iodine?

Nothing happened to iodine. Do you remember the skull and crossbones you once saw on iodine's labels? They meant it was poisonous if swallowed. It still is. "Iodine is quite toxic. You need to be careful about storing it far out of the reach of children," warns Jim Peters, Ph.D., pharmacy supervisor at the Oregon Health Sciences University Hospital.

What *has* happened is that faith in and use of iodine have declined. Once a staple of first-aid kits everywhere, it's now harder to find. Only a few products contain it. Should you, too, stay away from iodine? "Iodine is actually a fairly safe and effective drug if used properly," says Dr. Peters. Avoid using it on deep or large wounds. Some doctors think that it may irritate tissues, and inhibit healing in these cases. Also, it can cause allergic reactions.

Dr. Peters recommends you use products containing povidone-iodine (Betadine Ointment or Skin Cleanser). Povidone-iodine takes longer to work than pure iodine, because it is an organic compound. "The iodine has to become liberated from the povidone before it can become an antiseptic. But for minor wounds, delay won't matter. And povidone-iodine is less irritating to the skin. Plus, it's non-staining. If you're going to use it on a small wound that might then come in contact with your clothes, that's a real advantage," he says.

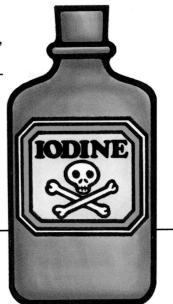

many useful, safe, nonprescription products are available now that self-care is not difficult. Read all labels, of course, and be aware of all precautions. But doing this—using over-the-counter products judiciously—is the smartest, least expensive and least painful approach to treatment that I know."

Sleep Aids and Wake-Ups

Sleep. Some nights, it can seem so elusive. Other times, it slips up on you when you don't want it to —right in the middle of a meeting, maybe, or during a long drive.

The result, this time, might be a slight swerve and a sudden wake-up. Next time, should you look in your medicine cabinet for relief from too little or too much sleep? Many of us do. We spend over $200 million yearly on over-the-counter sleeping pills alone. But can a good night's sleep, or a quick pick-me-up, come packed into a pill?

PILLS CAN MAKE YOU DROWSY

Many nonprescription sleeping pills use antihistamines as their active ingredient. Diphenhydramine hydrochloride is the most common (Sominex 2, Nytol, Compoz, Miles Nervine, Sleep-Eze 3); doxylamine succinate is another (Unisom). As sleep aids, both only recently became available without a prescription.

Of all the antihistamines, "diphenhydramine and doxylamine . . . are probably best suited for use as sleep aids since they have a highly sedative effect," explains Charles A. Walker, Ph.D., dean and professor of toxicology and pharmacology at Florida A&M University, Tallahassee.

In one study, doxylamine was shown to compare favorably to prescription sleeping pills; in another study, people who took the antihistamine fell asleep sooner and stayed asleep longer than those who took a placebo.

"All sleeping pills work by suppressing the entire central nervous system; they blunt your awareness physically and mentally," says Thomas Roth, Ph.D., director of the Sleep Disorders Clinic at the Henry Ford Hospital, Detroit, Michigan.

However, sensitivity to over-the-counter sleeping pills can vary widely from person to person, according to Dr. Walker. For unknown reasons, some of us just aren't affected when we take the pills at the recommended doses. If a sleep aid doesn't quickly make you feel drowsy, don't compensate by taking more pills. You could suffer toxic effects, Dr. Walker warns.

"Although the antihistamines have a wide margin of safety, potential poisoning . . . should not be discounted . . . especially if you take the pills in combination with alcohol," he says. Again, don't exceed the dosage recommended on the drugs' labels. Taking too many of the pills can actually *excite* your nervous system. And a wide-awake nervous system would be any insomniac's nightmare.

SOME PEOPLE SHOULDN'T USE SLEEPING PILLS

Avoid sleeping pills altogether if you have asthma, glaucoma, heart disease or are pregnant, urges Elliot Phillips, M.D., author of *Get a Good Night's Sleep*. And discontinue them if you develop dizziness, a dry mouth, blurred vision or constipation. All of these are side effects that may accompany antihistamine use.

Even if you feel no ill effects, don't rely on sleeping pills night after night, Dr. Phillips says. "They should be reserved for occasional use only, at times of increased stress or for . . . temporary conditions, such as jet lag."

Dr. Roth agrees. "Sleeping pills can mask serious physical or emotional problems," he says. "The only way to effectively treat insomnia is to find its cause. If you know the cause—say, marital stress—but can't live with your insomnia, ask your doctor about prescription sleeping pills to use for a brief period of time. However, if you *don't* know your insomnia's cause or if it continues for more than a week or so, sleeping pills aren't the answer, and you and your doctor will have to explore the problem further."

WHAT IF YOU CAN'T WAKE UP?

The flip side of insomnia is fatigue. In fact, many people who can't sleep at night find themselves fighting fatigue all afternoon. And many of these people rely on stimulants to ward off their drowsiness.

Caffeine is the only nonprescription stimulant available (No Doz, Vivarin, Efed II). Different brands contain different amounts of caffeine. Be sure to read and follow label directions about proper dosage.

According to the FDA, caffeine is a safe and effective stimulant when taken in doses of 100 to 200 milligrams, no more than every 3 to 4 hours. "In a study on driver performance, caffeine improved alertness," Dr. Walker reports. He also points out that, in other tests, caffeine improved typing, mathematical ability and puzzle-solving, especially when people were involved in those activities for a long time.

But another study found that, though people using caffeine *thought* they were more alert than before taking the drug, their actual performance on various tests was not improved at all. Caffeine can't sober you up, either. The only effect caffeine has on drunkenness, Dr. Walker says, is to make you less sleepy, but still drunk.

"Caffeine stimulants keep you awake. But you can still be woozy," Dr. Roth emphasizes. "The consequences can be serious, especially if you're driving. I wouldn't get in the car with someone using stimulants."

Heavy or long-term use of these pills, even if you're not driving, is never a good idea. "Small doses (50 to 200 milligrams) [may help] thoughts flow more easily . . . and fatigue decrease," Dr. Walker says. Larger doses can cause an array of side effects, including nervousness, headaches, irritability, rapid heartbeat and insomnia. You can also become dependent on caffeine.

"My advice if you have trouble staying awake during the day is to get more sleep at night," Dr. Roth says. "If you do sleep enough and still feel fatigued, see a doctor."

If you don't sleep well, the safest, cheapest, longest-lasting "medicine" may be a few simple changes in your lifestyle, according to Dr. Walker. Take a walk in the evening, don't nap during the day and try good, old, comforting warm milk before bedtime. With luck, you'll soon be sleeping better than a baby.

How Caffeine Pills Work

If you heed the dosage recommendations on either No Doz (2 tablets) or Vivarin (1 tablet), you'll swallow 200 milligrams of caffeine. You'll probably feel awake. But why and how? What is this much caffeine doing to you to make you feel so alert?

Caffeine provides a swift kick to your nervous system, according to Charles A. Walker, Ph.D., dean and professor of toxicology and pharmacology at Florida A&M University and contributor to the *Handbook of Non-Prescription Drugs*. Two hundred milligrams will immediately stimulate your adrenal glands to release adrenaline, a powerful hormone. As a result, your arteries contract, and your heart rate and breathing speed up.

But caffeine also *directly* stimulates the heart, making it pump harder and faster. In fact, more than 250 milligrams of caffeine can cause cardiac irregularities.

And while it's doing a number on your heart, it's not neglecting the other muscles in your body: It tightens them. That's one reason you feel more awake—and tenser.

Those stimulated muscles might come in handy, though—you'll probably have to walk to the bathroom a lot. Caffeine is a diuretic: It stimulates your kidneys to increase urine output. It also stimulates another part of your digestive tract—your stomach—to increase *acid* output. And that can mean nausea and indigestion.

The drug can also damage your sleep. In some people, as little as 150 milligrams disrupts normal sleep patterns. You'll have more dream-sleep and drift into rejuvenating non-dream-sleep later and for less time than is normal.

Because of all these effects, you should probably think twice (or 3 or 4 times) before you use caffeine pills, especially if you have heart or stomach problems or are pregnant. "It's a mistake to fight fatigue by indulgence in stimulants," Dr. Walker says, and he suggests that people rest if they're tired. What if you're tired *all* the time, even when you get plenty of rest? Don't look for artificial energy in caffeine pills. Call your doctor.

3

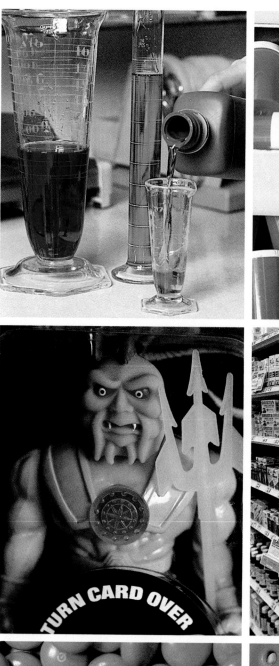

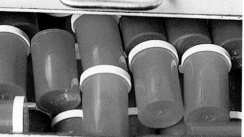

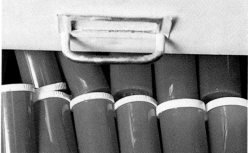

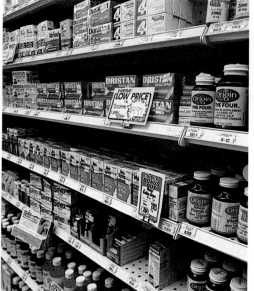

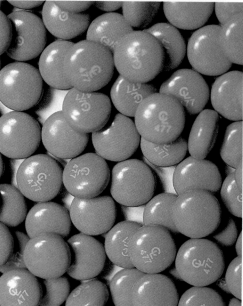

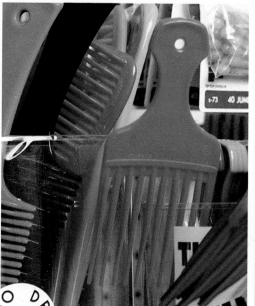

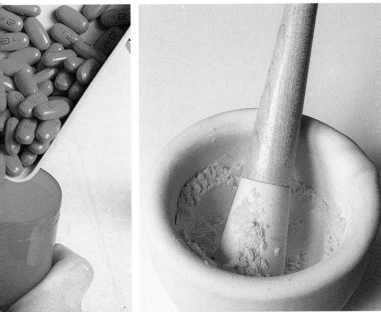

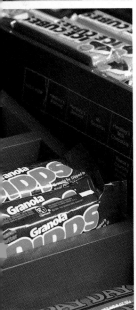

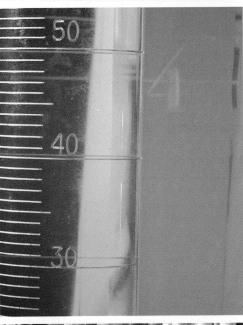

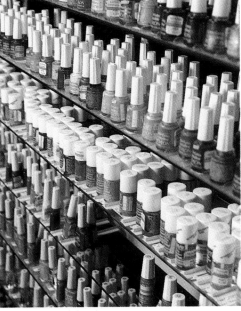

ION SHOULD BE
ITH PLENTY OF
ATER

MAY CAUSE
COLORATION
E URINE OR FECES

A FULL GLASS OF
GE JUICE or EAT
NANA DAILY
KING THIS MEDICATION

NOT DRINK
LIC BEVERAGES
g this medication

Inside Your Pharmacy

To get the best health care, choose a pharmacy as carefully as you would your doctor.

It seems that at the end of most visits to the doctor, especially if you have a specific health complaint, you are handed a prescription for a drug that will make you healthier, happier, sleepier, thinner, fatter, saner, calmer, or whatever you like. Armed with this official piece of paper, you may think that the diagnostic part of your illness is over and that it is time for the healing to begin. But there is still one very important place to visit: the pharmacy. You may think of the corner drugstore as quite ordinary, not much different from other stores. But it is a place of utmost importance. In fact, you should look at your pharmacy as the final stop on the road to good health. The pharmacist can explain instructions your doctor has given you about your medication, discuss any possible side effects, and catch any mistakes that might have been made when the medicine was prescribed (which are not as rare as you might imagine).

You probably fill several prescriptions a year; some people fill several a week. These drugs are important to your good health, but unless prescriptions are filled as they should be and the medicines taken correctly, they also can be very harmful. Careful preparation of drugs is just one good reason your pharmacist is so important.

Additionally, the pharmacist can provide the kind of day-to-day help you might hesitate to seek from your doctor, because doctors usually are so busy—and expensive. A good pharmacist, for example, can advise you about any over-the-counter drugs you are considering and whether they have any side effects.

The pharmacist as much as the physician is working for your life. Look at your pharmacist and pharmacy as health resources, and choose your drugstore as carefully as you choose your doctor.

THE FRIENDLY PROFESSIONALS

A pharmacy is nothing more than the sum of its parts—drugs, other items ranging from candy cough drops to bicycle patch kits, and the pharmacist. Without the last part, a drugstore is nothing more than a convenience store. But just what is a pharmacist, and what makes this person so important?

You walk into most pharmacies and see one or two people—women seem to be about as common as men these days—standing behind a counter, typing labels, peeling stickers and pressing them on bottles, stapling receipts to the folded corners of sacks and handing the packages with authority to a teenage cashier.

You see them pulling large bottles from shelves, counting pills and, just occasionally, mixing powders and liquids together to turn your bad health into good. Sometimes you'll see them fret and worry and dial a telephone. Is all this really anything special? Have you ever wondered what it is that makes a pharmacist a professional? After all, couldn't anyone with a high school education count pills and type prescription labels to stick on bottles?

Of course. But could anyone with a high school education understand the chemical makeup of thousands of drugs and countless combinations of these drugs? Could just anyone let you know when your doctor—that harried professional who seems to know almost everything but rarely has time to share it with you—has made a mistake?

Of course not. And that's why we have pharmacists. Pharmacists who are licensed by the state. Pharmacists who are well educated and highly skilled.

TEAM HEALTH: PHARMACISTS, DOCTORS, NURSES

These professionals, with their friendly, store-on-the-corner image, are as important to the health-care system as guides are to a national park. Without them we would be even more confused by all the health options available to us. We would have a much harder time finding our way around.

"Pharmacists are an integral part of the health-care triad, along with nurses and physicians," says William N. Tindall, Ph.D., director of professional affairs for the National Association of Retail Druggists in Alexandria, Virginia. "They know your health-care providers in town and provide you with an excellent entry point into the health-care system."

And the pharmacist isn't just a pawn in the doctor's game. "They are just as much professionals as any physician," says Dr. Tindall. "They are dealing with people's health just as much, if not more."

In fact, if the doctor makes a mistake in prescribing medication, the pharmacist must catch it or be held liable for damages. If, during the 1½ minutes your doctor spends diagnosing little Susan's cold, he prescribes an adult dose of medicated cough syrup, not noticing that she weighs only 45 pounds, the pharmacist must catch the mistake. It is the pharmacist's duty to call the doctor and remind him that such a large dose could be dangerous. If the doctor won't make the change, it is the pharmacist's obligation to warn you, or not fill the prescription. He would also be perfectly in line if he recommended that you take little Susan to a new physician.

Not all physicians' prescribing mistakes are due to negligence. Many result from a lack of time to keep up with current drug developments—a difficulty compounded by the physician's limited medical training in pharmacology.

Pharmacists are far more qualified than physicians to gauge the actions of drugs because they are better educated about drugs. Pharmacists average three full years studying pharmacology—the action of drugs in the body—during their five- to six-year professional education. A doctor usually spends only one or two semesters studying drugs. That's a big difference.

The relationship between doctor and pharmacist is similar to that of an architect and an electrician. While the architect is trained to look at the big picture (and, like the doctor, is

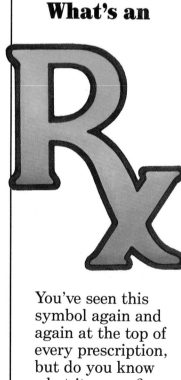

What's an

Rx

You've seen this symbol again and again at the top of every prescription, but do you know what it means?

Rx is an abbreviation of the Latin word *recipe*, which means "take."

well paid to do it), he might not be skilled in working out all the important, possibly hidden, details. While you would trust him to design a beautiful, functional house, you would certainly hope that he hires a competent electrician to make sure the house won't burn down due to faulty wiring.

DRUG SCORE: PHYSICIANS 25, PHARMACISTS 6,000

This difference in education and emphasis is also why physicians generally know the effects of only the 20 or 25 drugs they routinely prescribe. Physicians just don't have time to keep up with all the other drugs, because they have so much other medical information to sort out. But pharmacists do. It is their job to understand drugs. A competent pharmacist should know something about (or be able to find information immediately in a book) any of the 6,000 drugs that the average pharmacy stocks.

Pharmacists study biology, math, physics and chemistry in their quest to understand drugs. They learn about toxicity, metabolism and absorption of drugs—in short, everything about how drugs act in the body. They learn how to mix drugs and dispense them. And some schools teach their pharmacists how to deal with patients and help other professionals like doctors prescribe the best treatments possible.

This professionalism and sense of duty are necessary, because pharmacists aren't playing a game when they step behind the counter. Their job carries a lot of responsibility. "We've found that there is a potential for problems with drug interaction in 17 percent of new prescriptions that come across our counters," says Kenneth W. Anderson, a pharmacist, who is vice president and director of professional services for Medicare-Glaser Corporation, a large pharmacy chain in the St. Louis area. "Of those prescriptions with a potential for interaction, 5.7 percent are significant, requiring the pharmacist to call the doctor or counsel the patient on what the problem is. The others are more minor interactions

John H. Jones, M.D.
1000 W. State Blvd.
Anytown, USA 13468

Name _____

Address _____ Date _____

Phone: 555-1248
office hours by appointment

Reg. No. LIS-54630
DC7455018

Decoding the Mystery

Unless you've studied Latin, prescriptions are impossible to understand. Here's your own translation guide.

Latin	Abbreviation	Meaning
ad libitum	ad lib	freely, as needed
ante cibos	a.c.	before meals
bis in die	b.i.d.	twice a day
capsula	caps	capsule
gutta	gtt	drop
hora somni	h.s.	at bedtime
per os	P.O.	by mouth
quaque 4 hora	q.4h	every 4 hours
quater in die	q.i.d.	4 times a day
signa	Sig.	write on label
ter in die	t.i.d.	3 times a day
ut dictum	Ut dict., UD	as directed

that will only be a serious problem if more than a few are present. It also depends on the patient's physical state and age. The pharmacist must judge," he says.

"If a pharmacist makes a mistake, it can be very serious to the patient," says Dr. Tindall. But pharmacists must be doing a good job filling prescriptions. For several years they were ranked just behind clergymen as the most trusted people in America, according to Gallup polls. And in 1983, pharmacists took over the number one spot.

You, the patient, are the one who benefits most from this trustworthiness. Pharmacists have been shown to play a subtle yet vital role in helping you maintain your good health.

A recent survey by the U.S. Food and Drug Administration found that the majority of pharmacists go to extra lengths to keep their customers informed. A survey of 241 pharma-

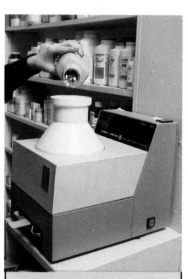

Pharmacy Services

Here's a checklist of services a very good pharmacy will provide.
• Patient's drug profile
• Computer check of drug interactions
• Generic substitutes
• Drug counseling; advice on OTC medication
• Educational pamphlets, stickers, books
• Itemized insurance and tax records
• Charge accounts
• Delivery
• 24-hour emergency service

cies in 23 cities in the United States and Puerto Rico showed that 97 percent use labels on their prescription drugs to remind the patient about side effects. Think about it: Would you remember which drugs not to take when you drive or which antibiotics shouldn't be taken with milk if your pharmacist didn't attach a label to the container? And 37 percent of the pharmacies surveyed also gave out leaflets that explained a drug's effects.

POSITIVE INFLUENCE

Studies have shown that the pharmacist's participation in the patient's health care plays a positive role in whether or not the patient takes the drugs according to directions (and gets healthy) or doesn't (and remains sick or gets worse).

Lawrence F. Nazarian, M.D., of the University of Rochester School of Medicine and Dentistry in New York, conducted a six-week study of patients and drug compliance (defined as taking at least 70 percent of a specific prescription as directed). He looked at 158 people who received prescriptions for antibiotics such as penicillin and ampicillin, which have to be taken faithfully for a period of time, usually ten days, to be effective. The patients were divided into three groups: Members of the first group got their prescription without any special instructions other than what was on the label and a brief sentence or two about how important it was to take the drugs as directed.

The second group, called the clock group, was given prescription bottles with a clocklike label on the front that told the patient the correct time to take the drugs. Plus, the pharmacist took extra time to explain the importance of compliance.

People in the third group, called the sticker group, were given basic instructions plus a large, bright red sticker with the patient's name, directions for taking the drug, and the day they should stop taking the drug, written on it. The patients were to stick the information on their refrigerator or medicine cabinet door. Again, the pharmacist took time to talk to the patient. The re-

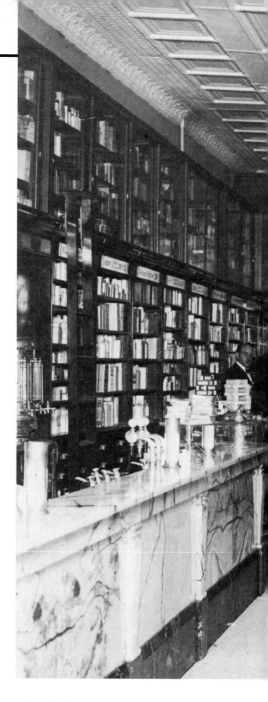

sults: Only 28 percent of the patients in the first group were compliant (took at least 70 percent of their prescription as directed); more than half (53 percent) of the clock group were compliant and fully 62 percent of the sticker group were compliant.

PERSONAL CONTACT IS THE KEY

When researchers questioned the patients later, they found that it wasn't the labels alone that led to increased compliance. Rather, it was the personal contact with the pharmacist as he explained the labels that made the biggest difference. The

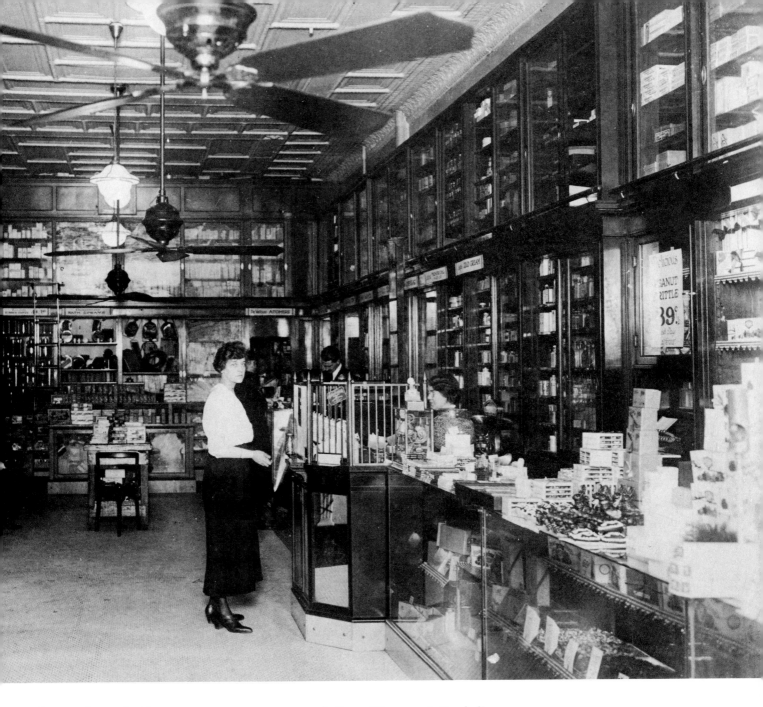

pharmacist probably spent no more than 2 to 4 minutes extra with each patient in the clock and sticker groups, but that little bit of time added a lot to the patients' health.

The lesson for you? Find a pharmacist who is willing to take the time to explain your drug therapy.

Additionally, make sure he not only explains it but also writes it out clearly, so you can understand it. "Effective patient instruction on how to take a prescribed medication obviously plays an important role in whether or not the therapy will have its intended results," according to the American Pharmaceutical Association, which has published a list of guidelines for pharmacists on filling

prescriptions. The association believes that you can get the maximum benefit from drug therapy with minimum side effects only if doctors and pharmacists work together to communicate with you. And, according to the association, the directions a pharmacist writes on labels "are critical to safe and effective drug therapy." You might want to check and see if your pharmacist supplies most, if not all, of the following information.

• The prescription label should contain the name, address and telephone number of the pharmacy; doctor's name; type and quantity of drug; directions for taking drug; date prescription was filled; number of refills; name of patient.

- Labels for potentially confusing drugs should say where the medication is to go—for example, drops for the nose or the eyes.
- Each label should have an expiration date, if one is needed.
- If a drug needs special storage, such as refrigeration, the label should say so.
- Any warnings, such as against driving while taking the medication, should be on the label or an adjacent sticker.
- In addition to writing a complete label, the pharmacist should give precise, concise *verbal* instructions on how to take the drug. If the pharmacist has any questions, the doctor should be called.

PATIENT PROFILES ARE ESSENTIAL

Obviously, finding a pharmacist who is willing to discuss your prescriptions with you is very important. But it is not the only important factor. Most people ask their friends' advice and do a little research before choosing a physician. You should do the same when selecting a pharmacy. And once you find one that you trust, stick with it. It is wise to keep all your drug information in one place in case of possible interactions between a newly prescribed drug and one you are already taking.

To prevent these problems, "Patients should look for a pharmacist who keeps patient profiles of medication," says Philip Oppenheimer, Pharm.D., of the School of Pharmacy at the University of Southern California in Los Angeles. Such a profile will include a list of any allergies, chronic illnesses, frequently used over-the-counter drugs, prescription medicine you are now taking and any other health information the pharmacist feels is necessary, such as your age and general well-being. The pharmacist can then consult this information when filling a prescription.

"The average patient sees more than one doctor—a specialist for his

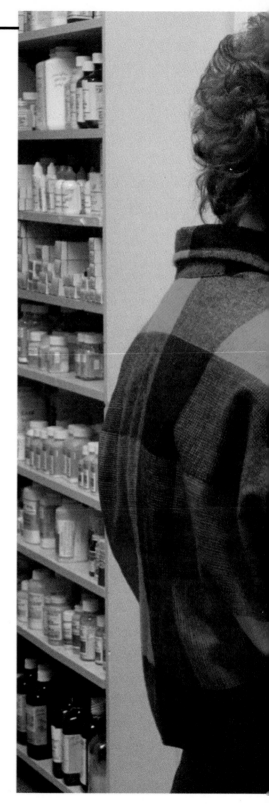

heart and another doctor for another problem—but 70 percent of people use only one pharmacy. This is important because doctors often do not communicate with each other. The pharmacist then assumes the role of having to determine if the drugs prescribed by one doctor are interacting badly with the drugs prescribed by another," says Dr. Tindall.

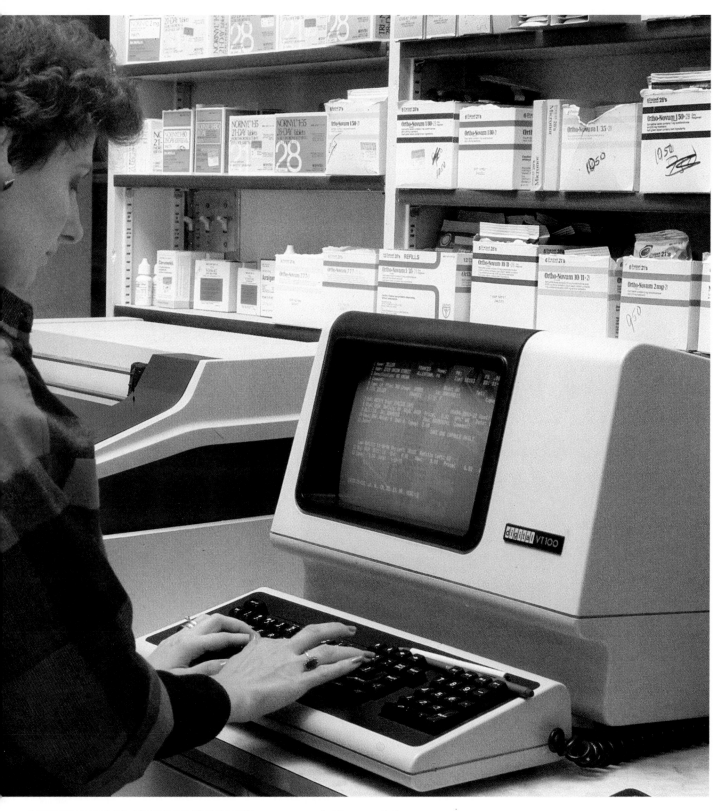

COMPUTERS SPOT PROBLEMS

Spotting these drug interactions can be a tricky process for even the most talented and brainy pharmacists, because there are so many possible drug combinations. There are an average of 2.5 chemicals in each prescription, and the average person fills between two and four new prescriptions a year. That's a lot of interactions right there. Add to that all the possible influences of over-the-counter drugs, allergies and diseases, and you have many potential problems. To keep track of all these chemicals requires a computer brain. Not too many people have this capability, so many pharmacies have turned to computers to give their customers better service.

"We have 11,500 interactions in our computer system, and no human could possibly keep track of all those," says Kenneth Anderson. His 100 stores all have small computers connected to a mainframe—a large computer in the home office that does all the work. "The computer speeds up the check for drug interactions and does it with a thoroughness that would not be humanly possible," he says. Each drug is screened automatically for three things: drug-to-drug interactions, drug-to-allergy interactions and drug-to-disease interactions. The system is effective: At least two or three problem interactions are noticed—and taken care of—by pharmacists in the stores each day.

And the machines apparently haven't upped the price of prescriptions at the chain's stores. "We have weighted the efficiency of computers and cost and found that because the computer allows efficient pricing, inventory, label typing and other services, it offsets the extra cost. In fact, we think we are more competitive now," says Anderson. So while a computer might not be an absolute necessity for a pharmacist, you might want to have your prescriptions filled at a store that is computerized.

Still, all the electronic memory in the world won't do you any good if you don't have a pharmacist who talks things over with you. Otherwise, the information will be about as useful as snowshoes in a desert. "People should have a pharmacist who takes the time to provide medication counseling—one who will tell the patient how to take the medication, how to store it, why it is being prescribed, what to expect from it and what side effects might occur," says Dr. Oppenheimer.

Of course, the pharmacist shouldn't be considered a social service to brighten up a dull afternoon. They are busy professionals. (One former employee of a friendly pharmacist remembers the small crowd that would gather around the counter in late afternoon, talking and asking the pharmacist questions. He finally had to put a stop to it, losing some

customers as a result. It was the only way he could get his work done). Still, if your pharmacist won't take the time to talk to you, spend some time looking for another.

HELP AT TAX TIME

Another thing you might look for is whether or not the pharmacist will keep track of your drug purchases, either with a computer or by hand. This service is important for your insurance records and taxes. Also, if you move to another town, you'll want to give your drug profile to your new pharmacist.

To get a copy of your prescription records, just ask your pharmacist. You have a right to a copy of them, though the original prescriptions become the property of the pharmacy when they're filled. While some pharmacies will submit bills directly to your insurance company, most won't, because it is not economical. So, when you are ready to send them in, just ask your pharmacist to give you an itemized account of your purchases.

This record also helps on April 15. If you need a list of your prescription drugs for the Internal Revenue Service, don't hesitate to ask your pharmacist. It might save you a big headache if you are audited. And if you travel, take a list of your current prescriptions with you in case any of your medicine is lost or stolen. This precaution is especially important abroad, where many medicines have different brand names than they do in the United States and a list of generic names might be handy.

THE GENERIC REVOLUTION

Drugs can be a big-ticket item. Many people who regularly take medicine are on fixed incomes and can't afford to spend much, even on their health. And even those few who aren't watching their pennies don't feel right paying higher prices than they have to. For all these people, generic drugs are a blessing.

Not too long ago a patient was

left in the dark when it came to drug prices. If your doctor told you to take a drug, you took it. And you paid whatever it cost. Now there is a popular new alternative to paying high prices, for some drugs at least. Generics are catching on. Yes, they are similar in some ways to the generic items you see in grocery stores: The all-white boxes with black lettering that tells you exactly what's inside without a lot of colorful, enticing graphics. Like store generics, the no-frills drugs are as good as the brand names, but less expensive because they aren't promoted. (Advertising has to be paid for by the consumer, just like everything else, so no advertising means lower prices.)

While some big drug manufacturers argue that generic drugs are inferior to name brands, their objections don't really hold up. According to the FDA, generic drugs have the same chemical structures as brand-name drugs; the generics just look different. For example, generic Valium (diazepam) doesn't have the same designer look as the product sold by the Roche Company—but it has the same mood-altering effect. In the past, makers of generic drugs had to submit detailed tests to the FDA to prove the drugs were safe, even though they were identical copies of drugs the FDA had already approved. Today the companies need to show only that their generic drugs are chemically equivalent to the brand-name products and that their products' therapeutic effects will be the same.

While new drugs usually are patented, many drugs have outlived their patent and thus can be copied by generic manufacturers. Drug patents expire all the time. So if any of the drugs you now take aren't yet available in generic form, chances are they will be in the next several years.

REFRESH YOUR DOCTOR'S MEMORY

You might have to do a little work to get a generic drug. While your pharmacist undoubtedly stocks most of what is available, some doctors routinely specify brand names. If

What to Do If Your Pharmacy Goes out of Business

Though pharmacies are usually stable businesses, they sometimes fail or close. Should you panic if yours goes out of business?

No. You won't have to visit your doctor again for new copies of your old prescriptions, you'll just need to find out where the old ones are. "Nine times out of ten, another drugstore will have purchased the files," says William N. Tindall, Ph.D., of the National Association of Retail Druggists. If you haven't been notified of the change and there is no sign on the failed pharmacy's door, call the state health department to find out who has your files.

Then, if you want to use the drugstore that purchased your files, they'll verify your prescriptions with your doctor at no charge and continue to keep your financial and medication records. If you want to use a different pharmacy, ask for a copy of your records and give them to the pharmacy of your choice. Remember, your prescription history is rightfully yours, at no charge, so don't hesitate to ask for it.

the doctor doesn't give his permission, the pharmacist isn't allowed to substitute the less costly generic drug. So any time you get a prescription from your doctor, or have an old one renewed, be sure to ask him to okay a generic substitution. If he won't, ask him why. He might have a good reason for not substituting drugs. If he doesn't, it might be a good idea to find a new doctor.

If your pharmacist refuses to provide a generic even when your doctor says it is all right, find another pharmacy. All 50 states allow pharmacists to use generics unless the doctor forbids it.

ADVICE ON THE DANGERS OF "SAFE" DRUGS

Along with providing information on prescription drugs, most pharmacists are qualified and more than willing to give you advice about over-the-counter drugs you take to treat yourself. You might be surprised at how potent some of these drugs are (see chapter 2) and how important it is to know what you are taking, especially when you are also taking other drugs. The Consumer Information Service of the National Association of Retail Druggists suggests that you should consult your pharmacist before purchasing any nonprescription medicines. The association says that the pharmacist "considers it among his most important professional services to discuss such matters with you."

Although your pharmacist certainly isn't qualified to diagnose and treat medical problems, the pharmacy is a great referral center. If you feel ill but aren't certain whether you should see a doctor or try to doctor yourself, approach your pharmacist for information. Chances are he will be able to recommend several good physicians you could see. Or he might suggest that you wait a bit to see if you feel better.

Other services to look for in a pharmacy include delivery and 24-hour emergency service. Delivery can be especially important to those who are unable to drive or get around well because of illness, or who just feel too miserable to get out of bed. Many pharmacies provide this service at little or no charge.

Twenty-four-hour emergency service also can be very helpful, though it isn't quite as common as delivery service. If your child wakes in the middle of the night with one of his recurring ear infections, you'll want to be able to fill his prescription for antibiotics and pain relievers so he—and you—can get at least a few hours of sleep.

Finally, a service pharmacies provide that you should be able to take for granted is confidentiality. "Pharmacists are bound to confidentiality, just like doctors, lawyers and psychiatrists," says Dr. Tindall, "so no one should worry that someone else will find out what kind of medicine they are taking."

WHAT KIND OF PHARMACY TO CHOOSE

Now that you know *what* to look for in a pharmacy, the next problem is deciding just *where* to look. There are many different kinds of pharmacies, all of which offer their own conveniences and drawbacks. Some are as noisy and busy as Fifth Avenue on the day before Christmas, while others are as quiet as Main Street on Sunday morning. Your needs will determine which type you choose. But remember, whichever pharmacy you pick, stick with it. It pays to have all your prescription information in one place. And it is comforting to know just who is filling those important prescriptions for you.

Years ago there was only one kind of pharmacy—the corner pharmacy—but these days big discount pharmacies seem to have a large share of the marketplace. These come in two main types, the store that calls itself a pharmacy but will sell you everything from goldfish to reflective cotton running shorts, and the discount department store that advertises reduced prescription and over-the-counter drug prices at the back of the store. Either store will net you one main benefit: low prices.

THE BATTLE OVER WHO IS BEST

These big discount pharmacies are usually part of large chains and the reason they can offer big savings is because they buy their drugs in bulk. They usually have several pharmacists working at a time and often seem impersonal. With the pharmacist hidden at the back of a store filled mainly with long aisles of shampoo, plastic picnic plates and silverware, hibachi grills in the spring and snow shovels in the fall, cigarettes and cigars, stationery and magazines, it is often hard to imagine that you are getting individualized service when your prescription is filled.

In fact, many chains require their pharmacists to meet a quota—they have to fill a certain number of prescriptions a day in order to justify their salaries—so it is possible that you will be brushed aside more quickly than you would like. All this provides a lot of fuel for the fires of criticism of chain pharmacies. "The chain pharmacists are under the gun and have less time to chat, to provide personal service," says Dr. Tindall

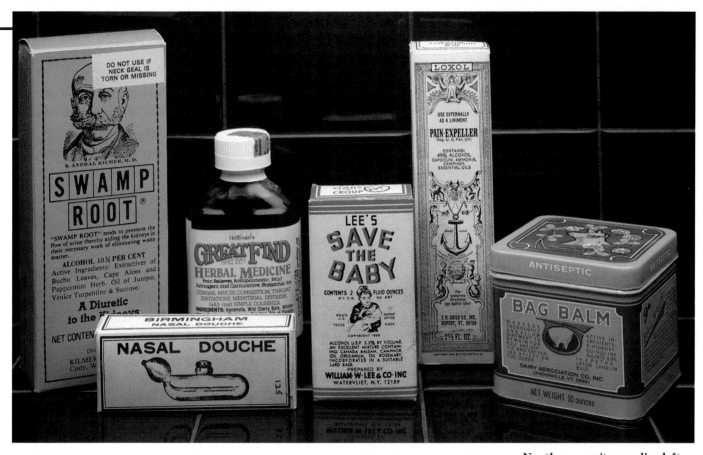

of the National Association of Retail Druggists.

"That statement is totally inaccurate," says Kenneth Anderson of the 100-pharmacy chain, Medicare-Glaser Corporation. "First, I've worked in both areas, with a chain and in a smaller, private drugstore. With the chain, all the administrative work, like ordering, pricing and paperwork, is done by others at the main office. That frees the pharmacist for counseling the patient. A small-time pharmacist has to do all that himself. We are very aggressive in getting information to the public."

But opinions are like pharmacies; they come in all types, and each has some merit. "The pharmacist in a smaller, community store counsels one-third more than a pharmacist in a chain store," says Dr. Tindall. He adds that this personal service means better service for you. "Pharmacists are often an integral part of the community. In small towns in Nebraska, North Dakota and elsewhere, the pharmacists often serve closely with the doctors and the hospitals in giving you the best health care." However, a small pharmacy might not have such modern and expensive-to-purchase services

as a computer to check your prescription for bad drug interactions. And the smaller store might not be open as many hours as the larger chain stores.

It is doubtful that the argument will ever be resolved by anyone but you. It's up to you to make the decision. If low prices are most important to you, try a chain pharmacy. You will no doubt get good service and good advice if the store is reputable. But if you want the feeling of walking into a smaller store where the pharmacist will know your name, then by all means have your prescriptions filled at a corner drugstore. Both are staffed by licensed, qualified pharmacists.

SEDATE, WELL ORDERED, PROFESSIONAL

While the above-mentioned pharmacies are the most visible, they certainly aren't the only choices for the consumer trying to pick the best. Still another type of pharmacy is the professional pharmacy. These aren't as common as other types— estimates are that there are only a thousand or so in the United States.

No, these aren't remedies left in the back of the medicine cabinet by Great-grandma Worswick before she went to that big liniment dispensary in the sky. They're products still sold today. The Bag Balm is really meant to soothe the chapped teats of milking cows, but some people put it on their hands. Lee's Save the Baby says it won't really save babies, just help them. Swamp Root is good for "flushing the kidneys," according to the label, and you could probably serve it at your next cocktail party along with the Pain Expeller—both are high in alcohol. The Herbal Medicine is "great" if you can "find" it. As for the nasal douche, don't laugh—there's no point in being too stuffy about old-fashioned medicines.

Their emphasis on patient education in a clinical setting, however, might make them the pharmacies of the future.

JUNK FREE

Eugene V. White runs an "office" pharmacy in Berryville, Virginia. Berryville is small, the kind of town where you'd expect the drugstore to have a long soda fountain serving cherry phosphates, banana splits and chicken salad sandwiches on toast. But White's pharmacy has no frills, not even greeting cards, candy bars, knitting needles, shoe polish, wrapping paper and ribbon, rubber cement, shoe sole inserts or sunglasses.

What the pharmacy does have is a clean, chest-high counter, two or three old-time pharmaceutical symbols hanging from the wall and an enclosed work area that removes the drugs from public view. It also has a small, private counseling room that is integral to White's philosophy. White will meet with a patient for free in this consultation room and answer any questions about drugs. If the questions concern a prescription that is being filled, there is an extra charge. And the patient is free to consult any of the books, pamphlets and audio-visual lessons that the pharmacy maintains to educate patients.

The basis of any discussion between White and a patient is the patient profile. This sheet lists all the necessary information about drugs and allergies and also lists the phone numbers of the patient's doctors. While these profiles are common enough now, White was one of the first pharmacists to recognize their importance. And you can bet that he makes extensive use of them.

Central to White's pharmacy is professionalism and a lack of commercialization. Choose this type of pharmacy and you will get the best attention, but you'll have to buy your shampoo somewhere else. Unless it's medicated.

POSTAGE PRESCRIPTIONS

At the other end of the pharmacy spectrum are mail-order operations. They offer the cheapest prices, convenience (the drugs are delivered right to your door with the mail) and some counseling. But they are remote.

Charles Byrne owns Pharmaceutical Services, Inc., in Belton, Missouri, outside Kansas City, but serves customers from all around the country. Missouri residents are his biggest customers, followed by people in California and Pennsylvania. The way it works is simple. People get their prescription from the doctor and mail it to the company. A few days later the medicine arrives in a shrink-wrapped (sealed in plastic) package that ensures the drugs haven't been tampered with. While this service isn't good in case of emergencies, it is useful for patients who regularly take specific drugs for chronic illnesses.

The mail-order pharmacy does have its advantages, along with the obvious drawback of being so remote from its customers. Foremost is cost. Mail-order pharmacies buy in bulk and have low overhead, so their prices are cheaper than even the discount houses. "If you belong to one of the groups that we sell to, such as a teachers' association, the price you pay will be lower than the price the wholesaler charges a drugstore," says Byrne. For patients who do not belong to a group, savings will average from 20 to 30 percent.

Byrne's company keeps patient profiles, just like a regular drugstore, and gives interaction information in the form of pamphlets and labels. If anyone has a question that needs an *immediate* answer, they can always telephone for advice.

By Byrne's estimate there are six or so mail-order pharmacies in the country. One of the largest is run by the American Association of Retired Persons. They fill millions of prescriptions each year from several locations nationwide.

GETTING THE MOST FROM A HOSPITAL PHARMACY

Finally, there is one type of pharmacy that most people don't take the time to choose: the hospital pharmacy. Even though people usually don't shop for hospitals, it might pay to examine their pharmacy services before the need arises, says Michael Stolar, Ph.D., director of scientific affairs for the American Society of Hospital Pharmacists in Bethesda, Maryland.

Dr. Stolar suggests that prospective patients speak to the pharmacy directors of local hospitals and find out if they offer these important services.

- Does the hospital have unit-dose distribution? Traditionally, a hospital pharmacy sends a bottle of medicine containing a week's supply of drugs to a patient's floor. The nurse then determines how much of the drug to administer and when to give it, based on written instructions she is given. This method can encourage error, because nurses have many patients and many drugs to cope with. Unit-dose distribution goes a long way toward solving dosage problems. With it, the pharmacist sets aside individually packaged and labeled doses in a drawer for each patient. They are placed in carts which are wheeled to the hospital floors each morning. With this system nurses only have to open a patient's drawer and take out the premeasured dose when it is time for the patient's medicine. Studies have shown that unit-dose distribution can reduce errors in drug administration by as much as 75 percent.

- Does the hospital have a clinical pharmacy program? This type of program has pharmacists visiting patients and checking medical records. The pharmacists, working with doctors, of course, would help the patient get the best drug treatment possible.

- Does the hospital have a strong formulary? The formulary is a system whereby a committee of physicians and pharmacists meets regularly to discuss drug effectiveness, the need for new drugs and the lack of need for out-dated drugs. The end result of these meetings is efficient drug purchasing and prescribing and lower bills for you.

Unfortunately, there is little you can do about high drug prices in hospitals other than tell your doctor to prescribe as cheaply and sparingly as he feels is safe. Hospitals with a formulary system don't stock duplicate brands or even every drug of a particular kind. They buy generically in the sense that they request bids on a given generic drug and then buy the cheapest form offered, be it a brand name or a generic equivalent. Thus, your doctor can't order you a cheaper generic substitution as he can when you go to a regular drugstore.

As you can see, there is a lot to think about when you choose a pharmacy—perhaps more than you ever imagined. But the little time spent choosing one will pay off in good health and good service for you.

4

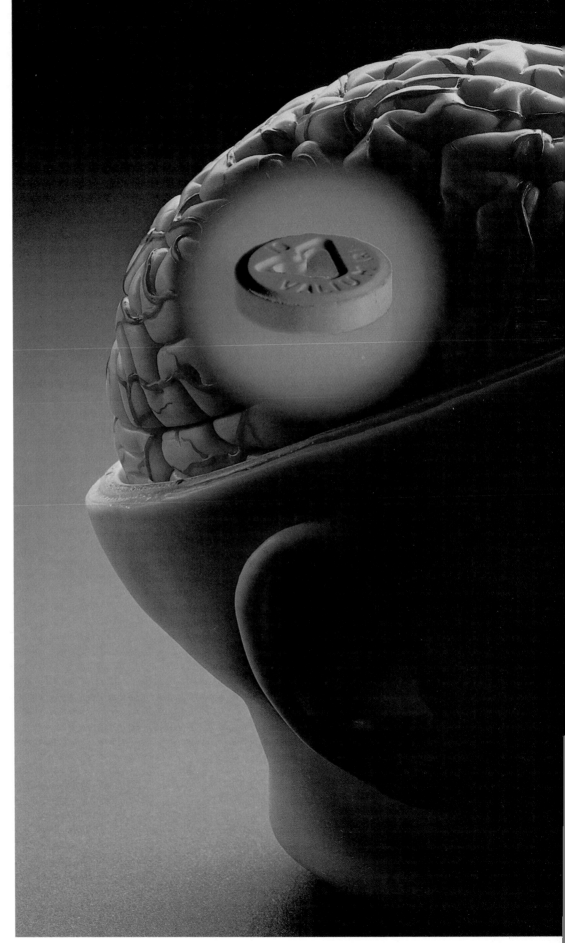

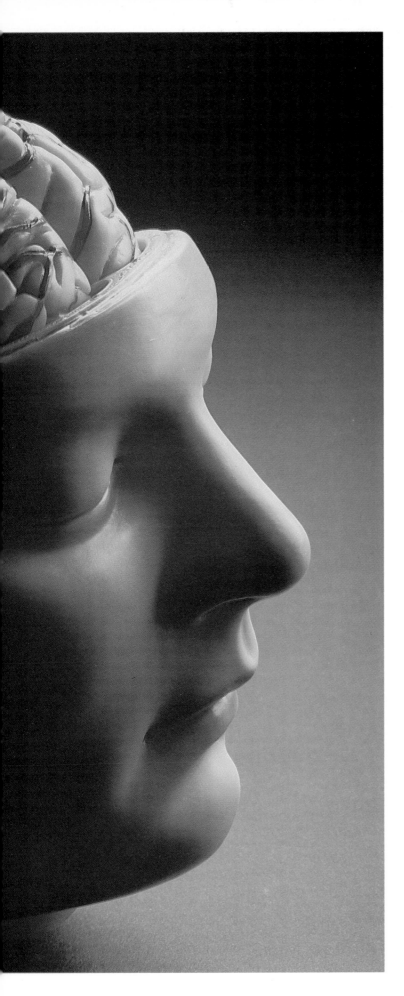

The Mind Drugs

They calm you down, speed you up, knock you out. They work. Just be sure you really need them.

An elderly woman's husband dies. For weeks after the funeral, she is sad but calm, a portrait of wise resignation, of quiet, abiding acceptance. But her strength is not so much from the Lord as from the pharmacist— she's taking the tranquilizer Valium.

A mental patient is discharged from the hospital and reenters the community. He works as a janitor for an insurance company, dutifully mopping the floors and cleaning the toilets. True, his smile seems oddly fixed and he continually talks to himself. But gone are the voices that spoke of a vast conspiracy to take his life; gone are the visions of purple lizards crawling in his shadow. Is he cured? No, but he's functioning— because he's on Thorazine, a so-called major tranquilizer.

Valium, Thorazine—two of a class of drugs that doctors call psychoactive and that we've labeled mind drugs. These drugs are controversial, to say the least. Some critics of Thorazine, for example, say it's a pharmaceutical straitjacket, a way to control the huge population of people with severe mental illness and avoid the time and expense of cure. Others say schizophrenics are better off sedated and sociable than violent and isolated. And Valium—is it a chemical crutch or a synthetic savior, a way to deny problems or a way to keep them at bay until the sufferer is strong enough to cope?

Hard questions. And equally tough questions could be asked about the use of antidepressants, sleeping pills and amphetamines. Who has the answers?

If a doctor prescribes a mind drug for you or someone close to you, it's *you* who has to decide if there's a real need. But to do this you need information, and that's what you'll find here. We tell you about the mind drugs—their dangers, drawbacks and disasters, but also their authentic usefulness in certain situations. And we start with the most common mind drugs of all—the minor tranquilizers.

THE SEDATION EPIDEMIC

They're called minor to contrast them with more powerful tranquilizers (which are called major, of course). But there's nothing minor about how much they're used. Take the scene in the Burt Reynolds movie *Starting Over*, for instance. The star suffers an anxiety attack in a department store. When a curious crowd gathers, his brother, Dom DeLuise, asks if anyone has a Valium. Purses fly open, pockets are searched, pillboxes snap wide: *everyone* does.

Valium use may never have been quite that epidemic, but this minor tranquilizer was the number one prescribed drug for eight years running.

In 1983, 25 million prescriptions of at least 55 pills each were written—that's almost 1.4 *billion* pills! And the use of Valium has actually *dropped*. Its peak was in 1975, when Roche (the American division of Hoffman La Roche, the giant Swiss drug consortium) sold almost 3.5 billion pills, or 15 pills for every man, woman and child in America.

What exactly is this drug? And why are so many people taking it?

Valium (or diazepam, its generic name) is one of a family of closely related drugs called the benzodiazepines that account for 85 percent of all minor tranquilizers prescribed in the U.S. They are most commonly used to treat anxiety and its symptoms, although they also have other uses, which vary according to the brand and the manufacturer.

Contrary to popular belief, a typical tranquilizer user isn't a hard-driving professional under extraordinary stress, but an elderly woman. Figures from the National Institute of Drug Abuse show that 42 percent of all American women have used tranquilizers, but only 27 percent of all men have. A poll published in *Science News* found that seven of every ten habitual users are over the age of 50, many of them widows suffering from chronic physical disorders and depression. Some suffer from Valium addiction.

THE "SAFEST" PRESCRIPTION DRUG?

Did we say Valium addiction? Yes, it's true: Valium can hook you, and as many as three million Americans have been at risk of addiction. And possible addiction is only part of the problem. A reporting system representing one-third of America's hospitals noted that 13,258 emergency room visits in 1982 involved the use of Valium, either alone or in combination with other drugs. Only alcohol provoked more emergency room visits.

Even more frightening, Valium was the fifth largest chemical killer in 1982, accounting for the deaths of at least 275 people—deaths caused by overdoses, nearly all in combination with other drugs or alcohol. The combination of Valium and alcohol is particularly dangerous because both depress the central nervous system. Together, in doses large

What Happened When Valium Was Banned?

Not prescribe *Valium?*

For most psychiatrists, that restriction would be the same as a ban on couches. But that's exactly what happened at the Naval Hospital in Long Beach, California, in 1976—a time when prescriptions for Valium were at their peak. What were the consequences when the tranquilizer (and its cousin, Librium) were locked out of the medicine cabinet?

"The patients feel relieved and say that they have for some time suspected that 'those drugs aren't doing anything,'" said a Long Beach study. "They are delighted by the dawning discovery that they can learn to manage their own lives, and that life is *not* a 'Valium deficiency.'"

"We've found that Valium is of very limited use here—on a *short-term* basis as a muscle relaxant and a tension and stress reliever," comments Theodore Williams, M.D., head of the Alcohol Rehabilitation Service/Substance Abuse Department at Long Beach. (The drug has since been okayed on a restricted basis.) "Its potential for abuse is just too great."

enough, they can stop breathing and produce coma.

Ironically, Valium is one of the *safer* mind drugs. John Doorley, assistant director of public relations for Roche, says, "Valium is one of the safest prescription drugs ever manufactured." What else would a PR man say, right?

Yet even its critics admit its safety. With proper use in moderate doses over limited periods of time, it's nearly impossible to overdose on Valium alone.

The benzodiazepines are, in fact, so effective in treatment of anxiety symptoms that they've been prescribed for just about anything from psychosomatic ailments to gastrointestinal complaints. That is the problem: They're *over*prescribed. The appalling statistics come not so much from its use as from its massive overuse.

"A major problem is that someone goes into a doctor's office and says, 'Doctor, I'm nervous,' and the doctor prematurely hands him a prescription for a tranquilizer," says Alan Schatzberg, M.D., associate professor of psychiatry at Harvard Medical School. "It's a disturbing fact that 94 percent of all tranquilizer prescriptions are written by nonpsychiatrists, yet it's psychiatrists who treat the truly serious cases of anxiety for which tranquilizers are truly useful," he says. "I'd say 18 to 20 percent are written for women by their obstetricians and gynecologists. The rest are written by primary-care physicians like internists, general practitioners, family doctors."

Not everyone gets Valium because they're uptight. The drug's other accepted uses are for the relief of the agitation, tremors and delirium of alcohol withdrawal; the relief of muscle and nerve spasm and pain; and as an anticonvulsant.

John Merritt, M.D., consultant for physical medicine and rehabilitation at the Mayo Clinic in Minnesota, said he prescribes Valium for spinal cord injuries (as well as nondrug therapies), for stilling the runaway reflexes that can result from brain and nerve disorders and for muscular and skeletal pain. Yet Valium is not always the best choice for some of

Valium Use Drops

Valium prescriptions are way, way down. Why? Because patients and doctors are far more cautious after the spate of Valium addiction stories. A recent survey of young Texas physicians showed that 40 percent believed that prescribing tranquilizers like Valium wasn't helpful and often made patients worse, even though almost half said that anxiety was more difficult to treat than most other medical problems. What's more, 67 percent felt their patients wouldn't suffer if the Valium family of tranquilizers (benzodiazepines) was removed from the market altogether!

these conditions. When the problem is primarily one of pain rather than muscle spasms, aspirin may be the best choice.

"I've seen studies that looked at aspirin compared to Valium and found aspirin was just as effective in relieving pain," Dr. Merritt says. "But Valium does make people more relaxed, and if a person's been injured and suddenly is confined to bed, he could get very restless. My personal opinion is that Valium is most useful in allowing a patient to tolerate bed rest better, but we certainly don't use it for more than two weeks."

Why the 14-day limit? Because Dr. Merritt is aware of the problem that can turn Valium from a gentle restraint on anxiety to a ball and chain shackled around your life: addiction.

SIGNS OF ADDICTION

And we're not talking about a bad habit, like eating ice cream after every meal. We mean real, physical addiction that can lead to withdrawal symptoms like soaking sweats, tremors, listlessness, painful sensitivity to sound and smell, insomnia, hallucinations, shakiness, seizures, convulsions, muscle cramps, nausea, vomiting and self-destructive behavior. A former Valium addict describes his withdrawal as " . . . if somebody pours kerosene over your skin and then every so often they touch a torch to it or set it on fire." And because it takes the human body so long to metabolize Valium, these withdrawal symptoms can set in anywhere from three days to five weeks after you quit.

Roche insists that addiction is very rare, occurring only because of patient overuse. Yet in a scientific study, 43 percent of patients treated for eight months or more with Valium showed withdrawal symptoms when they stopped the drug. After eight months of continuous use, the study said, withdrawal reactions occur with substantial frequency.

In other words, you don't have to take this drug for years to be at risk for addiction. One year is more than long enough.

PREVENTING ADDICTION

How can you prevent addiction to a minor tranquilizer? The most important thing is to take responsibility for your health. While you may have heard about problems caused by taking some well-known tranquilizers, you may be unaware that lesser-known, related tranquilizers can also cause problems. Therefore, don't let your doctor write a prescription for a drug you are unfamiliar with. If you don't know what it is, look it up in the *Physicians' Desk Reference (PDR)* or another drug manual. Ask your doctor to write a prescription for no more than 20 pills, which ought to last you a week, and to write "No Refill" on the prescription so you'll come back to discuss the drug's effects and won't be tempted to refill it the five more times the law allows.

It's important to know that there is *no* evidence that Valium or the other benzodiazepines are effective after four months of steady use.

At that point, the "relief" you feel when you take the drug may be nothing more than the fending off of the withdrawal symptoms that start to creep in as the drug wears off and that you now mistake for the original anxiety. In short, if you've been taking Valium or another benzodiazepine for a period of months or years, your body might be dependent on it. How can you tell? These are the classic signs of addiction:

- You feel you just can't function without it.
- You need more and more to get the same effect, and it fades more quickly.
- You've tried to quit but couldn't because the physical sensations were overwhelmingly negative.

If you have any of these symptoms, you may be addicted to your medication. Whatever you do, don't try to withdraw alone. Ask the doctor who prescribed the drug to help you.

VALIUM AND ALCOHOL: DOUBLE TROUBLE

If you think breaking an addiction to Valium is tough, imagine removing the hook of Valium *and* alcohol. Ironically, an alcoholic can get addicted to Valium *because* he's trying to dry out—Valium is used to treat the symptoms of alcoholics who are in the process of giving up drinking. Like so many other common uses of Valium, it might be the wrong drug at the wrong time. Researchers at the University of California at San Diego found that a group of rats on Valium favored alcohol more than a group of rats not on the drug.

But people aren't rats. Still, emergency rooms are visited by thousands of people who have done an alcohol/Valium whammy on themselves, and celebrities like Betty Ford and Liza Minnelli—to name just two—have publicly admitted dual alcohol and Valium addictions.

However, Colonel Carl H. Gunderson, M.D., head of neurology at Walter Reed Army Medical Center, says if the alcoholic patient is kept under strict observation and tranquilizer use is limited to a short period,

Valium and Librium (another benzo-diazepine) can work to stop DTs (delirium tremens). Yet he does admit that the doses needed to do this are much larger than doses the average person would ever be likely to take.*

ADDED SIDE EFFECTS

Valium's side effects don't end with addiction. So far, the list of suspected side effects of *normal doses* includes birth defects; memory loss; loss of coordination; changes in the level of sexual desire; so-called paradoxical reactions (the exact opposite of what the drug is supposed to do) like depression, acute anxiety, tremors, vertigo, hostility, excitement, aggression, delirium, rage or panic; swelling of breasts and milk flow in both sexes; drowsiness; fatigue; constipation and incontinence; headaches; high blood pressure; jaundice; skin rash; and blurred vision.

Even Roche admits Valium is hazardous in pregnancy, when taken with alcohol or other drugs and when taken during activities requiring high degrees of manual dexterity and coordination, like driving.

One study of young Dutch policemen given Valium showed significant loss of driving skill. And this was in their own patrol cars, on stretches of highway they were thoroughly familiar with!

Is there a way to take Valium and not end up in a head-on collision with bad news?

Valium and other minor tranquilizers are strikingly effective at temporarily reducing anxiety, but they cannot remove its source.

Too many people have used them as a way to pave over life's rough spots when at best they are a temporary bridge to psychological therapy (if the anxiety is serious) or to a readjustment of lifestyle (if the anxiety is minimal). To use another metaphor, diazepam can put you on the ladder to mental health, but it can't make you climb; you have to

*The opinions or assertions regarding treatment at Walter Reed Army Medical Center are the views of the author and are not to be construed as the official view of the Department of Defense or the Uniformed Service University of the Health Sciences.

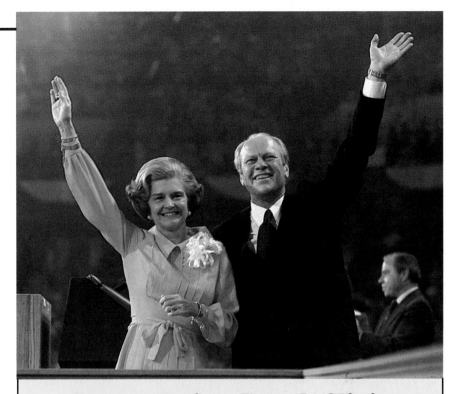

Former Patient Founds Clinic

Betty Ford had been on medication since the early 1960s for a pinched nerve, arthritis and muscle spasms, but the former First Lady never admitted she had a problem with addiction until after her husband left the White House. "So my speech had become deliberate," she wrote in her autobiography, *The Times of My Life.* "So I forgot a few phone calls. So I fell in the bathroom and cracked a few ribs."

Two days after her 60th birthday, Mrs. Ford entered the Alcohol Rehabilitation Service/Substance Abuse Department of the Naval Regional Medical Center, Long Beach, for dual addiction to Valium and alcohol. Eventually, she stopped both drugs, and once fully recovered she began investigating means to help others with drug problems. In October 1982, the Betty Ford Clinic in California was opened to help people with chemical addiction.

The program takes 5 to 6 weeks and family participation is mandatory. Only patients without severe medical or psychiatric problems are accepted, and—because hospital facilities are modest—the cost of a stay is extremely low.

"Mrs. Ford's talks and articles have helped enormously," says Susan Stevens, a spokesperson for the clinic. "People are beginning to look at the use of drugs and realize that it's not necessary to use tranquilizers, sleeping pills and painkillers for an extended period of time."

move your legs yourself. If you must, take it for a few days. After that the drug may take you—over.

THE HEAVY-HITTING TRANQUILIZERS

Valium is a weapon against anxiety, but compared to the major tranquilizers it's like a rifle next to an ICBM. The major tranquilizers are more dangerous but also strikingly effective. They can treat illnesses previously thought incurable, like acute schizophrenia and mania. It is these drugs, in part, that have caused the population of mental hospitals to drop precipitously from a high of more than 500,000 in 1955 to 132,000 in 1980. (And it's probably just as well. They weren't hospitals, but literally madhouses, filled with the ravings of violent patients in straitjackets, attendants built like halfbacks and the omnipresent odors of urine and excrement.)

Yet the decline is not without its critics, who charge that patients have just traded hospital confinement for the confinement of a drugged body. It's called the chemical straitjacket, and directly results from the use of major tranquilizers or antipsychotic drugs such as Thorazine, Stelazine, Mellaril, Prolixin, Haldol and Triavil. For better or worse, they have revolutionized psychiatry.

The discovery of drugs that can calm the most violent patients was one of this century's major developments in pharmacology. The historic treatment of the mentally ill in bedlams and so-called snakepits, which included whippings and frequent cold baths—torture, actually—gave way to experimentation with drugs in the 19th century. In World War II, doctors treating shell-shocked soldiers found some antihistamines to be wonderfully effective in calming them and cheering them up. After the war and into the 1950s, several research projects began the race to develop the first specifically antipsychotic drug, and Thorazine was introduced to the United States in 1954.

There is no question that antipsychotics do calm patients. Some 125 comparative studies to date in the United States alone show this class of drugs to be more effective than a placebo 82 to 100 percent of the time, a rate no other mind drug can claim.

HOSPITAL VS. COMMUNITY

When patients are "cured" with major tranquilizers, they often are released into a community that may be unprepared to receive them. Worse, there is no guarantee they will continue to take their drugs. As a result, they may end up back in the institution. A conservative estimate

---

Lecithin and Choline: Natural Help for a Severe Side Effect

Tardive dyskinesia (TD), with its spasmodic tics and grimaces, is probably the most startling side effect of any antipsychotic drug, but it need not be permanent. Researchers say choline—and lecithin, the substance from which it comes—may control it permanently.

Psychiatrists and physicians have long suspected that TD is actually the result of a deficiency in the brain of a chemical called acetylcholine. This chemical is a neurotransmitter responsible for the smooth functioning of nearly every part of the central nervous system. Choline (found in soybean lecithin, liver, eggs and fish) apparently is converted into acetylcholine.

Doctors at the Massachusetts Institute of Technology gave oral doses of choline to 20 TD victims and were very impressed by the results. TD noticeably diminished in 9 of them. Despite this test's success, there is one noticeable drawback to taking choline directly: It makes people smell like rotting fish. Fortunately, researchers at the University of Missouri in Columbia treated patients with lecithin rather than its single effective component and all improved—without smelling like a school of dead haddock. The Missouri scientists suggest lecithin might promise a permanent cure.

puts the return rate on patients who stop taking their drugs at 45 percent.

Why do they stop taking the drug that controls their disease? A Chicago professor of neurological sciences is quoted as saying, "People like diazepam (Valium), so they continue to take it. They don't like phenothiazines (major tranquilizers), so they don't take them for long." In fact, they're not even on the government's list of abused substances: Their effect is so unpleasant that the possibility of abusing them is zero.

TARDIVE DYSKINESIA AND OTHER SIDE EFFECTS

And there's certainly a lot to dislike. Anyone who's visited a loved one in a mental institution can tell you about patients in ill-fitting blue or green gowns wandering aimlessly like ghosts, some with faces and limbs horribly distorted and trembling uncontrollably, others rigid and apathetic.

It's even worse for the inhabitants, living with a florid psychosis that fills their days with confusion and terror—or being medicated with tranquilizers so powerful they can cause a serious, perhaps irreversible, disease that makes the tongue roll or dart, lips pucker and smack, eyes blink as rapidly as 40 times a minute and limbs twitch and shake like a rag doll's.

This horrible disease, called tardive dyskinesia (TD), is just one of the many side effects on a very long and ugly list.

Estimates have been made suggesting that half the patients taking major tranquilizers may suffer from tardive dyskinesia. TD was completely unknown before the mid-1950s but is now coming into prominence as one of the most stubborn neurological disorders ever seen. The evidence seems to be incontrovertible: TD is a disease created by the use of the powerful mind drugs.

Other suspected side effects of the major tranquilizers include lowered blood pressure that has resulted in death in some cases, elevated pulse, constipation, diarrhea, liver damage,

---

A Drug That Blows Your Cool

Summertime, when the livin' is easy—easy if you're not over 60 and on drugs like Thorazine, that is. Some 60 to 70 percent of all cases of heatstroke and 80 percent of heatstroke deaths occur in people over age 60, according to James Lipton, Ph.D., professor of physiology and anesthesiology at the University of Texas Health Science Center at Dallas—where they *know* about heat. Dr. Lipton also says antipsychotic drugs taken by older people can lead to heatstroke.

Older people's physiological responses have slowed with age, Dr. Lipton points out, so they might not be able to tell how really hot it is, and they won't sweat as easily. As a result, core body temperature shoots up. Thorazine compounds the problem even further by interfering with the body's "thermostat," leading to heatstroke.

What can you do? Dr. Lipton offers the following commonsense guidelines: Stay out of the heat, drink lots of water and avoid overexertion and alcohol.

---

hormone imbalance and impairment of the sex drive.

Jonathan Cole, M.D., co-director of the affective disease program and chief of the psychopharmacology program at McLean Hospital, a private hospital near Boston that is connected with Harvard, says, "Almost no one likes them. But psychotherapy alone is almost completely ineffective in schizophrenia and the acute manias. These drugs are so much better than nothing. It is a trade-off because of the side effects, but I wouldn't give patients dangerous drugs that could cause TD if they weren't really necessary."

DON'T BE RUSHED

If a doctor or psychiatrist recommends antipsychotics to you or to a loved one, remember they could work miracles—or cause permanent damage. And remember that patients have a right to refuse these drugs—a right that has been upheld by the Supreme Court.

Although there is no clear-cut therapeutic time frame, being on these drugs for the rest of one's life is a real possibility. Be particularly alert for severe side effects. If signs of TD develop, discuss with the doctor the possibility of alternatives, or at least a reduction in dosage.

Fortunately, few of us have to be treated with antipsychotics. But many of us, nevertheless, are exposed to one particular type of mind drug—sedatives used to treat insomnia.

30 MILLION TICKETS TO DREAMLAND

Lying awake, watching the digital minutes flicker into hours, is an infuriating experience for us and not an unusual one. Insomnia is the third most common reason Americans visit a doctor, right behind the common cold and headaches.

To get us to the Land of Nod, we use almost 30 million prescriptions for sleeping pills every year. (Many of those 30 million prescriptions are written for older people, even though they make up less than 12 percent of America's population.) These pills—doctors call them sedative-hypnotics—induce a calming, drowsy effect (sedation), hopefully leading you to fall asleep promptly, and promote sound sleep for some period of time (the "hypnotic" effect).

Actually, none of us should be overly concerned with the amount of sleep we get—or miss. Experts say it's not the *amount* of sleep you get but how you feel during the day that determines whether you have a problem. If you writhe in a tangle of sweaty sheets during the night but your day goes just fine, there's no need to treat for insomnia, says sleep expert Frank Zorick, M.D., medical director of the Sleep Disorder Research Center at the Henry Ford Hospital in Detroit. "It's only when insomnia becomes a problem of daytime functioning and performance that it should be treated," he points out.

But what if insomnia *is* fogging your brain? Sleep researchers have identified three major types of insomnia and determined whether or not sleeping pills can treat them.

THE THREE FACES OF A SLEEPLESS EVE

Transient Insomnia. This type causes the vast majority of sleepless nights. It's brought on by short-lived anxiety or changes in the body's circadian (waking and sleeping) schedule—changes like jet lag, new-job jitters or moving. Sleeping pills can work well for this type of occasional insomnia. However, if your job demands very high levels of alertness, you might be better off not taking them because of their "hangover" effect.

Short-Term Insomnia. This type of sleeplessness can be treated by hypnotics, too, but only for about three weeks. It is brought on by more serious anxiety, like the type caused by the death of a spouse.

Long-Term Insomnia. Deep emotional and physical problems that no pill can cure cause this kind of insomnia, which drags on week after week, month after month, year after year.

If your insomnia doesn't vanish when the pressure slacks off, you could have a genuine medical or psychological problem preventing you from getting the sleep you need. If such is the case, sleeping pills are only a Band-Aid for a profoundly deep wound. Here, the cure is treatment for the underlying problem.

What if your doctor can't find any problem that could cause your insomnia? Are you stuck with endless half-awake nights and half-asleep days? Not at all. Ask your doctor to refer you to sleep clinic. The specialists there will run complete physical and psychological exams, including interviewing your sleeping partner. If these exams aren't enough to pinpoint the problem, the specialists will monitor your vital signs while you sleep in the lab, interpret them, and make recommendations to your physician and you.

No matter which type of insomnia you have, if your doctor prescribes a pill it will probably be from the benzodiazepine family, the same class of drugs used to treat anxiety. The most frequently prescribed drugs in this group include Dalmane, Restoril and Halcion.

Before these drugs were developed, people took either barbiturates or any one of a variety of sleep-inducing concoctions, including thalidomide (which is almost synonymous with birth defects) and chloral hydrate (just a few drops of this sprinkled in a drink produced the original, sometimes fatal, "Mickey Finn").

Barbiturates are as effective as benzodiazepines in the short run, but they have some major disadvantages. Not only are they very addictive, but an overdose can be fatal. Also, barbiturates can combine with other substances that also depress the central nervous system (like alcohol) to produce lethal results. Barbiturates, in fact, caused 84 percent of all drug-related suicides or deaths by accidental overdose in the mid-1950s. After the introduction of benzodiazepines, however, barbiturate-related deaths dropped to less than 10 percent of such deaths in 1982, the last year for which statistics are available.

"The barbiturate hypnotics have been rendered obsolete by pharmacologic progress and deserve speedy oblivion," sermonized the *New England Journal of Medicine*. Dr. Zorick and William Sterling, Ph.D., senior associate director of clinical research at Sandoz, Inc., the drug company that manufactures the popular sleeping agent Restoril, agree that this group of drugs eventually will disappear entirely from medicine cabinets.

If your doctor prescribes a barbiturate, ask him why he isn't prescribing a milder sleeping pill. But be aware that even they can pose a risk.

NOT WITHOUT PROBLEMS

Death by overdose of benzodiazepines alone is almost impossible. But—just like barbiturates—they can cause death when taken with large doses of alcohol or other central nervous system depressants. Because benzo-diazepines are eliminated much more slowly from the body, after one week of continuous use they can accumulate to six times the level you started out with. If you drink heavily after taking them for a week or more, that "one for the road" could be for the road to the emergency room.

Another drawback is that some sleeping pills stop working after about a month. A study from Pennsylvania State University, reported in *Modern Medicine,* showed that sleeping pills' effects wore off after two weeks' use, making the user increase the dosage and leading to a spiraling effect that *worsened* the insomnia. (Six follow-up studies by the same doctor confirmed it.) If the person keeps taking pills, he may become addicted, experience worse insomnia *and* be groggy throughout the day.

Early studies of benzodiazepines were bursting with enthusiasm: They caused no barbiturate morning "hangover," they didn't cause early-morning awakenings, they didn't suppress the rapid-eye-movement (REM) stage of sleep that's associated with dreaming. Later studies questioned these early findings. Moreover, the new studies found another disadvantage: The benzodiazepines not only affect the REM or dream stage of sleep, they also disrupt later stages. "Benzodiazepines suppress the unique electrical brain activity associated with stage 3 and stage 4, or deep sleep," says Dr. Zorick. It's not known which of these stages is essential for rest, he says, but what is known is that you can wake up feeling just as tired from the benzodiazepines as from the barbiturates.

Getting a good night's sleep without the use of drugs isn't impossible. It takes time and medical attention, but it can be done. A study from the Stanford University School of Medicine involving a group of women showed that simply talking to the doctor every week, or using techniques like group therapy or meditation while gradually reducing the dosage, got most of them "unhooked" in six weeks. A follow-up study 18 months later showed most were getting 6 to 7 hours of good sleep every night.

Sleeping Pills, Broken Bones

Sure, sedatives make you fall asleep, but they just might make you fall down the stairs, too. A study of 75 patients at a veterans' home in California found that those who took sedatives were wobblier on their feet, more confused and fell more. And a British study showed that an amazing 93 percent of elderly hospital patients who suffered broken thigh bones at night were taking barbiturates.

It's not just that barbiturates can leave you as punch-drunk as a boxer in the 15th round; barbiturates also may actually lower the amount of calcium in the bloodstream by interfering with the absorption and utilization of vitamin D, which is essential for the absorption of calcium. Result: softened bones that break under stress.

FIGHTING DEPRESSION

Sir Winston Churchill called it his Black Dog. When young Congressman Abraham Lincoln got it, he'd take off to the woods. Thinkers from theologian Martin Luther to naturalist Charles Darwin had it, and artists ranging from Handel to Hemingway and Shelley to Presley were afflicted.

Ten-Gallon Health

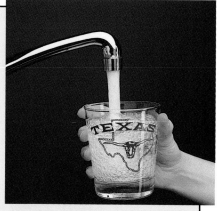

Q. What mineral is present in the water of western Texas?
A. Lots of lithium.

The above exchange is not from the game "Trivial Pursuit"—and the effect of lithium may not be trivial either. Consuming lots of this mineral appears to be linked with lower admission rates to mental hospitals. (Lithium is a natural mineral salt that doctors use as a drug to treat manic-depression.

Biochemist Earl B. Dawson, Ph.D., of the University of Texas, reported a significant relationship between the level of lithium in a community's drinking water and the rate of mental hospital admissions. It seems the higher the level of lithium in the water, the lower the rates. El Paso, in Texas's Western Panhandle, for instance, has one of the highest lithium levels in the Lone Star State. It also has about three times fewer psychiatric admissions, according to Dr. Dawson.

It's been rumored that Dr. Dawson is so enthusiastic about this link that he actually may have proposed putting lithium in community drinking water to keep us all smiling.

Some mental-health specialists who have studied this issue believe this idea is far-fetched and based on limited research. It seems we may never have the opportunity to try the drink that seems to make our Lone Star cousins so sunny.

The disease is severe depression, a condition that may be suffocating up to 15 million of us. One estimate puts a man's chances of being severely depressed at least once in his lifetime at one in ten and a woman's at one in four.

So-called normal depression is actually a period of recuperation following a setback. It's when the smothering pall doesn't lift for months, or deep despair and over-jubilant optimism alternate with pinwheel rapidity (a condition called manic-depression), that depression becomes a medical and psychiatric problem. At that point it's often treated with the class of drugs called antidepressants.

These drugs work by lifting the terrible weight of sadness or futility from the person who is depressed. Alexander Nies, M.D., professor of psychiatry at Dartmouth Medical School and an expert on these drugs, says, "They are not really mood elevators except in depression. When people who aren't depressed take them, very little happens." But if you are actually suffering from depression, they provide relief.

Actually, there are several kinds of antidepressant. One of them is called an MAO inhibitor. (This type includes Nardil and Parnate.) True, it sounds like an anticommunist Chinese commando, but it's really a compound that slows down the way the brain uses a chemical called monoamine oxidase (MAO), which scientists believe may cause depression by becoming too plentiful. Other types of antidepressants work differently and include the natural element lithium, the so-called tricyclics such as Elavil, Tofranil, Sinequan, Adapin, Asendin and Ludiomil, as well as combinations of antidepressants and tranquilizers, like Limbitrol.

These drugs are a fairly recent addition to a psychiatrist's black bag, and they work very well. One study of 1,300 severely depressed patients showed that 62 percent improved dramatically when given antidepressants. And in a Canadian study of 26 patients who didn't get better with one type of antidepressant, 24 were clearly improved within 48 hours of taking lithium. And when two patients were taken off lithium because their symptoms had disappeared entirely, they became depressed again within two days, according to reports in *Medical Tribune*.

But perhaps the biggest benefit of these drugs is that they improve depression faster than nature alone could. Alan Frazer, Ph.D., associate professor of pharmacology at the University of Pennsylvania, Philadelphia, points out that before the advent of antidepressants, 60 percent of all depressive patients improved in one year and 85 percent in two years. Most specialists agree that it takes about three to six weeks of antidepressant therapy to achieve a marked improvement.

"Antidepressants tend to get people out of a depression much quicker than if it's left to be treated by time alone," says Dr. Frazer. "If a member of my family were depressed and I had the choice of six weeks or two years, I'd take six weeks." Yet, a Johns Hopkins Medical School survey of almost 2,000 people in a western Maryland community revealed that very few individuals with symptoms of severe depression were taking antidepressants. Instead, many were taking Valium, which may deepen a sense of despair. Another study of 217 depressed people showed that barely 13 percent took antidepressants. Among those who did, doses were so low they probably had very little effect.

ANTIDEPRESSANTS AS A ROADBLOCK

The reason so few people suffering from depression are treated with antidepressants is that doctors are reluctant to prescribe them. True, they nuke depression. But they also produce fallout. Patients taking lithium, for example, have complained of feeling leaden, disassociated from their bodies and sometimes even more depressed. And MAO inhibitors taken in combination with certain other drugs, foods, cigarettes or alcohol can cause disastrous side effects, including one from which no one recovers: death.

The drug Asendin provides a glaring example of why doctors and psychiatrists are so cautious with

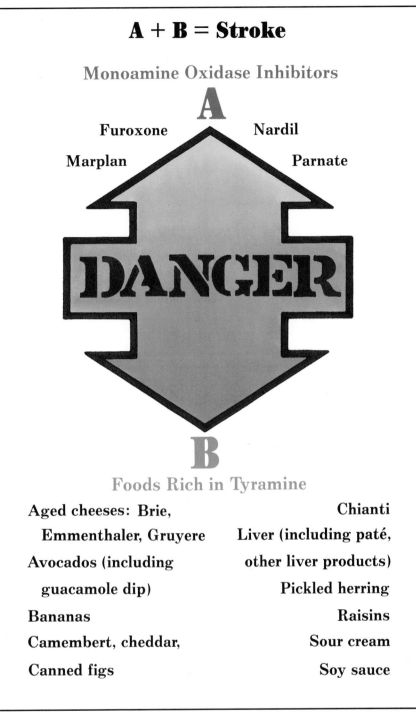

A + B = Stroke

Monoamine Oxidase Inhibitors

A

Furoxone   Nardil

Marplan   Parnate

DANGER

B

Foods Rich in Tyramine

Aged cheeses: Brie,	Chianti
Emmenthaler, Gruyere	Liver (including paté,
Avocados (including	other liver products)
guacamole dip)	Pickled herring
Bananas	Raisins
Camembert, cheddar,	Sour cream
Canned figs	Soy sauce

the antidepressants. This fairly new drug was introduced in 1980 with promises of fewer side effects and greater safety. By 1983, however, regional poison control centers in New Mexico and Washington, D.C., noted that people who took an overdose of Asendin had a death rate of 15.2 percent (compared to 0.7 percent for all other antidepressants) and that 36 percent had seizures.

Side effects from these drugs are much more pronounced in older patients. Unlike the side effects of the major tranquilizers, however, most

Your doctor may have told you, but we'll tell you again: Never, ever mix monoamine oxidase inhibitors (list A) with foods rich in tyramine (list B). Tyramine by itself raises blood pressure, but that action normally is blocked by monoamine oxidase (MAO), a chemical in your body. But MAO inhibitors do just that—they inhibit or stop its effect, allowing tyramine to go on a rampage and cause a potentially fatal rise in blood pressure.

of these vanish after treatment has been discontinued.

So what should you do if your doctor or psychiatrist recommends an antidepressant? Before taking the drug, ask whether you might experience any side effects. If the answer is yes, ask which will require immediate attention and which may fade in time. Doctors also recommend that you keep alcohol to a bare minimum —no more than one drink a day, if you must drink at all.

If one of the unwanted side effects is sedation, ask your doctor if the drug you're taking is one which can be taken in a once-a-day dosage, at night. If such a dose is possible, the sedation will occur when you are sleeping and therefore won't be likely to trouble you.

"SPEEDY" RELIEF

Amphetamines. Never has a type of drug been introduced with such enthusiasm and embraced so fervently by doctors and patients alike, only to plummet into utter disrepute.

The amphetamines include the original Benzedrine and Dexedrine, along with the more recent amphetaminelike drugs such as Cylert, Ritalin, Tenuate and Preludin. They promote a sense of euphoric, all-encompassing energy and confidence, but may cause severe depression once their effects wear off. Someone abusing them long enough may become psychotic, wildly paranoid and uncontrollably violent, have hallucinations and engage in bizarre, compulsive behavior.

Amphetamines, or speed, as they're aptly nicknamed, were first marketed as a cold and hay fever remedy, but athletes, students and scientists soon discovered the Benzedrine inhaler was good for a heck of a lot more than unclogging a stuffed-up schnoz. A Depression-era study conducted in Los Angeles noted that 67 percent of the volunteers felt euphoric and 62 percent felt a dramatic increase in confidence. Word spread quickly: The Wonder Drug is here.

Almost all the major powers used amphetamines in World War II to help their soldiers combat fatigue.

One of the reasons the German blitzkrieg was so successful may have been that their soldiers were cranked up on speed. And amphetamines were so abused in postwar Japan than an epidemic of unparalleled violent crime along with record hospitalizations for psychosis swept that country in the late 1940s and early 1950s.

Abuse mushroomed in the United States, too. College students cramming for finals and truck drivers on tight schedules thought speed was the greatest thing since all-night diners. Hippies liked the high, too, until they realized that speed's fast trip was one-way. "Speed Kills" became a slogan of the 1960s.

It's no wonder that accepted clinical uses of amphetamines have shrunk dramatically. A 1946 report listed 39 uses. Now there are only 2: treatment of narcolepsy, a chronic sleep disorder characterized by an irresistible urge to fall asleep, and treatment of attention deficit disorder (ADD) in children, otherwise known as hyperactivity.

While amphetamines can help in weight loss, at least seven states have drastically restricted their use because of potential side effects and the dangers of abuse.

A spokesman for the FDA said the agency had studied 10,000 cases of attempted weight loss with speed and found it effective for a maximum of two weeks. Any doctor who prescribes speed to you for weight loss is giving you an instant solution and ignoring the hard facts of calorie intake, metabolism and genetics.

The myth that speed enhances intellectual performance was perpetrated by early research in the 1930s and 1940s. At best, these drugs mask fatigue and improve performance at simple, repetitious tasks like sorting mail.

TWO LEGITIMATE USES

What narcoleptics need is to keep awake—and thus this group may benefit from amphetamines. The American Narcolepsy Association says as many as 200,000 Americans might have this condition. A narcoleptic may drop off to sleep even when engaged in something as interesting as sex, or injure himself or get fired from a job for seeming lazy and irresponsible.

Amphetamines combined with antidepressants keep the victim awake, but just as in weight control, the effect wanes rapidly.

Some doctors think amphetamines also help rein in unruly kids. Everyone loves a mischievous child, but when he ricochets off the walls in a nonstop screaming, destructive tantrum, parents and teachers don't think it's at all cute. Instead, they may turn to Ritalin to help this hyperactive child. By a paradoxical effect scientists still don't fully understand, Ritalin—an amphetaminelike drug—calms children down, enabling them to concentrate and lead more normal lives.

An Ohio pediatrician studied the effects of Ritalin on the non-academic abilities of 50 children suffering from attention deficit disorder. Ritalin and a placebo were given alternately every few weeks. Of the 50, 38 showed definite improvement in the kind of activity requiring sustained attention, greater dexterity and coordination. Some improved basketball skills while others settled down to religious instruction.

Like grown-ups, children also can suffer the drug side effects of insomnia, amphetamine psychosis, hallucinations and uncontrollable tics.

As with all mind drugs, the choice—to use or not to use—is yours. All of them have risks, sometimes serious ones. But all of them may also provide a way out of a tough situation that you no longer have the energy to deal with. Talk to your doctor frankly, weigh the alternatives, and if you do decide to use one, do so mindful of the cautions and warnings we've mentioned here.

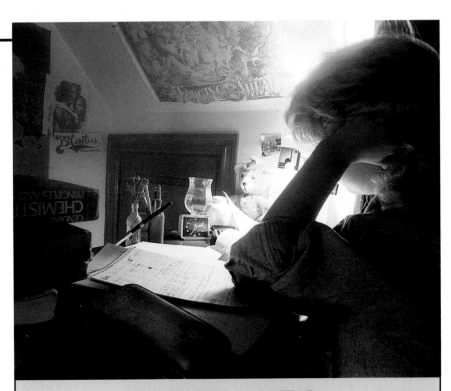

Speed Doesn't Help Students Think Fast

$S_1 + S_2 = A$; a simple and elegant formula college students have sworn by for almost half a century. If you stay up all night studying (S_1) on speed (S_2), you'll be in such tip-top form that excellent grades (A) come rolling in. Too bad that formula doesn't really add up.

It's true that amphetamines keep you awake and may improve short-term memory, but when it comes time to spit out what you've learned, you may be doomed to duncehood. The mistaken belief that amphetamines put your brain in fifth gear was started by a British test way back in 1936. Researchers gave 67 people amphetamines and discovered their scores on IQ tests rose an average of 8.7 percent. What they failed to mention was that 54 of these people were psychiatric patients. Later tests on amphetamines' effect on intelligence showed students taking the drugs did slightly *worse* than usual on reasoning tests, and did absolutely terrible on more complicated tests like arranging anagrams (the ancient Greek game of shifting letters from old words to make new ones). Tested hours after taking the drug, their problem-solving abilities were even more impaired.

Speed is close to being an anagram for stupid.

5

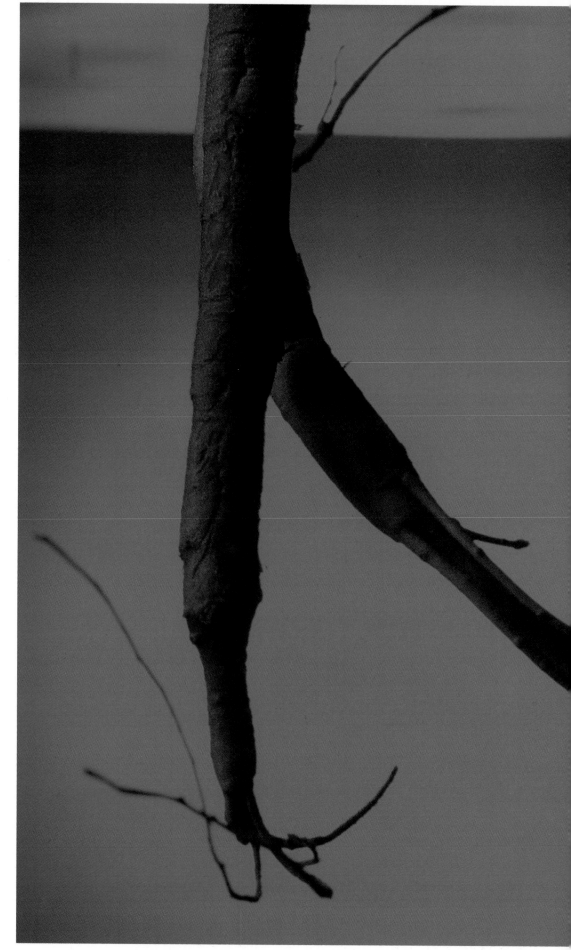

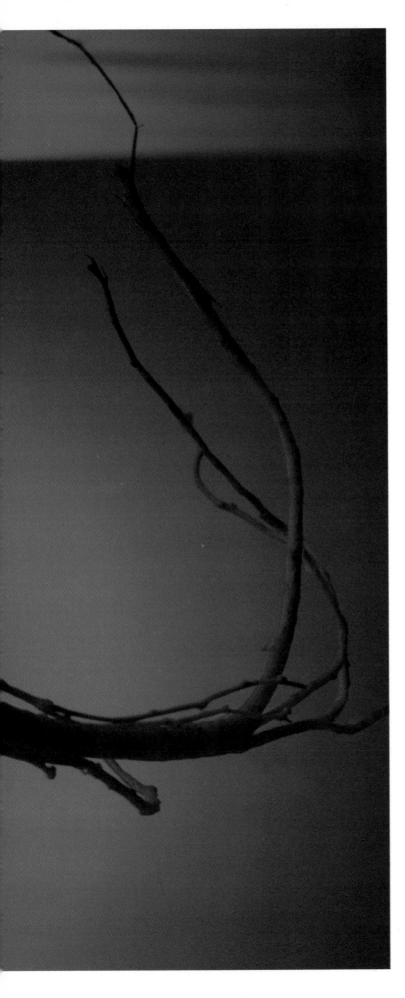

"Drugs" at the Health Food Store

An enticing alternative—healing substances that are not drugs. And not always safe.

Confronted with a growing list of dangerous side effects—or maybe just a growing amount owed to the local drugstore—you might be tempted to turn away from pharmaceuticals and instead place your hopes in the curative powers of herbs like ginseng (shown at left), or vitamins and minerals.

At such moments of temptation, it's not unusual to hear opposing arguments ringing in your mind. One little voice urges you to resist temptation—calling up the awful newspaper articles about people becoming sick from vitamin overdoses. The other voice nudges your thinking back to the health food store by promoting the theory that if these substances are "natural," they can't possibly be harmful. The fact is, neither of these arguments is especially valid.

Vitamins, minerals and even herbs are complex substances that can affect the human body in a variety of ways. While many have been found to be therapeutic for a variety of health conditions—for example, calcium to prevent osteoporosis, vitamin A to cure night blindness, vitamin B_6 for relief of carpal tunnel syndrome, vitamin C for the common cold—their very effectiveness clangs an alarm in the medical community. If these substances are strong enough to prevent or cure disease, the reasoning goes, they also may be strong enough to cause harm.

In fact, the use of vitamins and minerals to treat various diseases is considered to be so controversial that the U.S. Food and Drug Administration tried to regulate them in the same way that it regulates drugs. Twice. It failed both times.

Now simple common sense tells us that vitamins and minerals are necessary for good health. Taken in normal amounts, they don't require FDA approval or your doctor's okay.

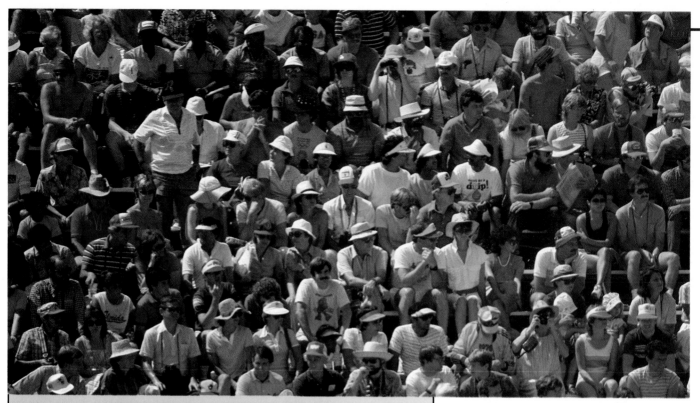

Who Takes Vitamins?

Picture the average vitamin taker. If your image was anything other than a college-educated career woman with a household income of more than $30,000, your view of vitamin users needs updating, according to a recent Gallup poll.

The poll also revealed that the approximately 60 percent of the adult population who take vitamin supplements tend to be—not surprisingly—more health-oriented than nonusers. Vitamin takers are less likely to smoke and more likely to eat wisely and to exercise.

Medical self-reliance also distinguishes the supplementers. They trust their ability to treat their own minor complaints like colds and sore throats, according to an FDA survey.

Glowing health, not just the absence of disease—that's what supplement users seek, the surveys show. And they get it, they say. Up to 80 percent report getting the results they want and feel good health is a good bargain for an average expenditure of a dime a day.

Nobel prize winner Linus Pauling, Ph.D., says, "You should no more consult a doctor before you take a vitamin than you consult a doctor before you eat some potatoes and carrots. Besides," he adds, "the doc-tor would probably give you the wrong advice."

Nevertheless, some controversy about almost every vitamin and mineral still exists. Troubling news reports appear frequently enough to generate distrust about their therapeutic value in the mind of the general public. Let's take a look at some of the claims and counterclaims.

CAN VITAMIN E CAUSE THROMBOPHLEBITIS?

If a vitamin could file suit for slander, vitamin E would seem to have a good case.

Since 1978, one doctor (and apparently only one doctor) has repeatedly raised the unconfirmed, unsubstantiated specter of health risks from vitamin E in daily doses as low as 100 international units (I.U.). First in a letter to the British medical journal *Lancet* and later in other publications, a doctor in private practice described a laundry list of symptoms he claimed to have seen in people who took vitamin E supplements. These ranged from chapped lips to leg cramps, from hypertension through sore breasts to thrombophlebitis.

It was a very odd list. At first glance, the symptoms and diseases on this list would seem to be helped— not caused—by vitamin E. In the words of James L. Baker, Jr., M.D., "Vitamin E is used specifically for the treatment of these exact disease entities."

The complaining doctor's main charge (repeated in letters to various medical journals in succeeding years and picked up by dozens of newspapers and magazines), was that vitamin E causes thrombophlebitis. This disorder is a painful inflammation of the veins associated with blood clots; its most famous sufferer was probably Richard Nixon. Thrombophlebitis is a particularly worrisome condition because of the possibility of clots breaking free and traveling to the heart or brain.

Some surgeons have used vitamin E to treat a variety of health conditions, noting that although vitamin E was not used to *treat* thrombophlebitis, blood clots rarely formed during this therapy. Some researchers are also convinced it helps to keep the veins from narrowing, a condition that can bring on thrombophlebitis.

SAFE—BUT SOME CAUTIONS

Is vitamin E safe when used as a supplement? The National Institutes of Health concluded that vitamin E in doses up to 400 I.U. daily has no harmful effect on people who take the vitamin on their own without consulting their doctor and without considering any other treatment their doctors may be giving them. The institute, in other words, says that vitamin E is safe to take, with or without your doctor's permission. However, there are two types of people who should begin taking vitamin E slowly—no more than 100 I.U. daily, some doctors advise.

People with high blood pressure should begin their dosage gradually. Why? "Vitamin E strengthens the heart muscle," says Samuel Ayres, M.D. As a result, contractions are stronger and blood volume greater with each beat. Dr. Ayres has recommended E to his patients for more than 25 years without ever seeing a problem caused by it.

Diabetics, too, should start with

a similarly modest dose. Research has shown that the vitamin may improve glucose tolerance, thus the diabetic may need less insulin. Without careful monitoring—which should be medically supervised—a diabetic might take more insulin than actually required.

Why has only one doctor witnessed any problems with vitamin E? No one has an answer to that question—other than one man's error.

SEX AND THE SINGLE VITAMIN

How did that rumor about vitamin E improving potency get started? Maybe it was because one of the first benefits of E to be discovered was its ability to help pregnant rats carry their litters to term and bear live young. Or maybe it was the studies on the fertility of white leghorn chickens.

The sex lives of rats and chickens aside, a deficiency doesn't seem to affect the human reproductive cycle. However, there are hopeful indications that E, because of its antioxidant properties, may slow the aging process.

But improving the frequency and duration of male erections? Unfortunately, that is wishful thinking, say doctors—though some benefit may be obtained from *believing* that vitamin E will work.

SHOULD A AND D BE GRADED F?

Vitamin A, the stuff of smooth, healthy skin, bright, sharp eyes and general glowing health, is poison. Or so you could easily believe if you paid attention only to newspaper stories about this nutritional component of beef liver, carrots, sweet potatoes and other foods.

Even though science has linked taking vitamin A with having better health, a longer life span, lower incidence of disease (including cancer) and greater ability to handle environmental pollution, the biggest headlines about vitamin A seem to relate to poisonings.

Is it possible to make yourself sick with vitamin A? Yes, it is. The

Safe Limits for Supplements

Unless you have specific reasons (and orders from your doctor) for taking large doses of vitamins or minerals, the limits below are good and conservative guidelines to follow.

Maximum Daily Dosage:

A—25,000 I.U.
Thiamine (B1)—25 mg.
Riboflavin (B2)— 25 mg.
Niacin—50 mg.
B6—50 mg.
B12—25 mcg.
Folate—800-1,200 mcg.
C—1,000 mg.
D—500 I.U.
E—600 I.U.
Calcium—1,200 mg.
Chromium—200 mcg.
Iron—30 mg.
Magnesium—400 mg.
Selenium—200 mcg.
Zinc—35 mg.

73

danger comes from overdosing, although you'd probably have to take 50,000 I.U. every day for a year to do it. Keep in mind that the maximum suggested supplementary level for vitamin A is 25,000 I.U. a day. Take that amount or less and everything's fine. Take more and there's a problem with potential overdose. The reason it's possible to take too much vitamin A is that it is fat soluble and can be stored in the body. Other fat-soluble vitamins include vitamins D, E and K.

Like practically every other substance on the earth, vitamin A can be harmful if too much is taken.

Quite surprisingly, the most serious vitamin poisonings seem to have occurred not from taking supplements, but rather through the misuse of foods. Among the handful of deaths resulting from an overdose of vitamin A were those of Arctic explorers who, against native advice, ate polar bear liver, a food containing massive amounts of the vitamin.

In less exotic situations, children have accidentally been overdosed on fish-liver oil and, in one case, on chicken livers. Twin baby girls became nauseated and irritable after eating chicken liver twice daily for several months. Their discomfort apparently was the result of too much vitamin A rather than mere dietary displeasure.

According to the *New York Times,* a few other unfortunate children given doses of A up to 100 times the adult Recommended Dietary Allowance (RDA) have also suffered serious discomfort—headaches, nausea, dry, cracking skin, bone pain and temporary injuries to liver and kidneys. But a sensible diet and supplement program will bypass these problems.

Vitamin D, the sunshine vitamin made by our skin, the preventer of rickets, can also be overdone, in supplemental form. In 1928, a scientist first noted that rats given cod-liver oil—the very thing that saved their lives when added to a nutritious diet—suffered hair loss, weight loss, diarrhea and eventual death when the oil was given in huge and excessive quantities.

Again, because D is fat soluble and therefore builds up in the tissues, people obviously should not take amounts that are greatly in excess of the RDA, which is 400 I.U. a day. Too much vitamin D can cause an overabundance of calcium to be released into the bloodstream, resulting in hypercalcemia.

When a Vitamin Becomes a Drug

Vitamins, whose very name suggests health and well-being, are probably one of the last things you'd think of when someone says "drug."

But psychiatrist José Yaryura-Tobias, M.D., thought "drug" when he considered vitamins' possibilities. In experiments with hundreds of patients, he and other physicians have tested massive doses of vitamins as druglike treatments for a number of serious illnesses from schizophrenia to mental retardation.

"A vitamin becomes a drug when I use it to try to alter and manipulate the body's chemistry," explains Dr. Yaryura-Tobias.

One of his theories grew out of vitamin B_6's role as a coenzyme or catalyst in the conversion of one brain chemical to another. Dr. Yaryura-Tobias hopes that in *large* doses B_6 can change that conversion in a way that helps relieve certain symptoms of mental illness.

"When vitamins are used in these amounts, they may even cause side effects like drugs," says Dr. Yaryura-Tobias. Self-dosing with B_6 in large quantities could cause neurological damage, he says, which is why no one should use large amounts of vitamins without their doctor's approval.

DOES VITAMIN C EAT B_{12}?

Chemist Martin Marcus was at a party when he first heard of the scientific report saying that vitamin C destroys B_{12}.

His first thought was of his wife, who had been taking 2 grams of C a day, and he was worried. "Oh, my gosh, I thought, she's going to get pernicious anemia," he later recalled.

He vowed to test a sample of his wife's blood for signs of the emergence of the dreadful disease. Pernicious anemia is caused by a lack of vitamin B_{12}, which the article had suggested that taking C could destroy. When he tested his wife's sample, Marcus was relieved to find no sign of any deficiency disease. He was relieved—but puzzled. "That was the first clue," said the chemist, who worked at Lincoln Hospital in the Bronx, where he now heads the chemistry lab.

Marcus tried to repeat the experiment that was first conducted by Victor Herbert, M.D., a longtime critic of what he regards as the unnecessary use of vitamin and mineral supplements.

But Marcus's result contradicted Dr. Herbert's. Vitamin B_{12} did not disappear when it was brought into contact with C. It was a scientific mystery. Marcus looked again at Dr. Herbert's test. What had happened? How had Dr. Herbert obtained his results?

The answer was simple, says Marcus. Apparently a crucial step had been left out of the standard procedure of the day—a step that would have protected the B_{12}. The lost step explained the lost B_{12}. The deficiency existed only in a test tube, not in the bodies of people taking vitamin C.

Thus C remains an immensely useful supplement—one that even Dr. Herbert admits may relieve mild cold symptoms.

THE GREAT DOLOMITE DEBATE

Because the common sea-made mineral dolomite contains two key human nutrients, calcium and magnesium, it has been used for years as an inexpensive supplement by people who wanted to make sure they got enough of both.

But in recent years, some supplement users became frightened of using dolomite. Fear-provoking articles appeared in newspapers saying dolomite samples had been found to contain possibly harmful levels of toxic metals, including lead. Many people who needed the added minerals stopped taking them.

Perhaps significantly, the same physician who claimed that vitamin E causes thrombophlebitis is a major character in the dolomite debate.

This doctor seems to have been the first to question dolomite's safety.

In a letter to a medical journal, he reported seeing "health-conscious patients" with "neurologic and other disorders." He suspected their disorders were the result of toxic metal poisoning from the supplements they were taking, he said. Therefore, he analyzed a sample of dolomite, only to find dangerous levels of lead. Although he refused to reveal the name of the company that had allegedly marketed the dolomite, newspapers around the country nevertheless reported that lead had been found.

MORE BAD PRESS

Later, the *New England Journal of Medicine* printed a letter charging that both dolomite and bone meal, another cheap, natural source of calcium and magnesium, might contain toxic metals. Again, newspapers gave the information wide play. The U.S. Food and Drug Administration also acted to test dolomite and bone meal for toxic metal content, and their announcement that some supplements had been found to contain lead and other dangerous metals also got wide play in the press.

What almost no one mentioned was that lead is found just about everywhere, since the metal is naturally present in the environment. The key question is, of course, do dolomite and bone meal contain a hazardous amount of metal?

Tests of samples done by three independent labs failed to turn up dangerous amounts of lead or any other toxic metal in the dolomite and bone meal supplements. What they did show, in fact, was that the nonhazardous amount of lead we consume daily is 35 times as great as the amount found in three average supplement tablets.

It's lucky that these two supplements are safe to take, because to get our daily requirement of calcium from milk would mean an extra 340 calories in addition to the extra money we'd spend. Ironically, that amount of milk would contain an equal—and equally safe—amount of lead as that found in the "dangerous" dolomite and bone meal.

B₆—TOO MUCH OF A GOOD THING

For years, vitamin B₆ (pyridoxine) got nothing but good publicity. It seemed that evidence mounted daily of some new condition this jack-of-all-trades vitamin appeared to help. From acne and Chinese restaurant syndrome (oversensitivity to a common ingredient in Chinese food, monosodium glutamate) to the very painful carpal tunnel syndrome, B₆ seemed to bring relief.

Because it is especially esteemed for its help with menstrual symptoms, some people even nicknamed this vitamin "God's gift to women."

But suddenly B₆ showed up as a villain in the press. A neurologist, Herbert Schaumberg, M.D., had found women with ducklike walks—"broad-based and stamping," as he put it—and a loss of sensation in their extremities. Extremely large doses of vitamin B₆ were the cause. The unfortunate distinction of being the first water-soluble vitamin shown capable of bringing on significant physical problems went to B₆.

Seven women out of the estimated millions taking the vitamin had suffered ill effects from consuming daily quantities of *not less than* 500 times the RDA for periods of months and years. Since that initial discovery, 40 more women with apparent B₆ overdose syndrome have been found. Although some people have taken the same amounts for long periods without ill effects, this practice is now considered unsafe.

Why were these women taking such massive quantities of B₆—2 to 6 grams a day—for months and years? Three of the original seven victims were doing so on the advice of their doctors. Why these doctors were unaware of published articles in medical journals describing the dangers of B₆ overdose is unclear. The other four women had self-prescribed B₆ for water retention or simply as a diet supplement. In at least one case, the woman kept increasing the dose, attempting to get the desired results.

But no woman who has experienced the miraculous improvement a small amount of B₆ can produce in her monthly menstrual symptoms is likely to stop taking it. Nor need she.

This vitamin is as safe as the bananas in which it is found. But just as you wouldn't eat 100 bananas in one day, you also should keep your vitamin intake at a sane level. And if you are planning to take B₆ or any vitamin in an attempt to

---

Muscle Pills Lack Strength

"Runners' Formula," "Athletes' Pack," "Super Energy Complex," "Muscle Power Tabs"—vitamin, mineral, protein and amino acid combinations such as these are offered to exercisers in ads that seem almost to promise Olympic gold in one swallow.

Alas, the experts say you can't dose yourself into greater distance or pill your way to a better performance. Any "suggestion that a product could increase athletic ability" is "false," according to the U.S. Food and Drug Administration.

Not that athletes don't need more nutrients than their desk-bound peers. Actually, they do—from the obvious need for more calories to the rather subtle requirements for increased iron and potassium and added B vitamins.

In other words, deficiencies can harm athletic endeavor. But athletes who are getting all the nutrients they need won't improve their performance by taking extra. Prepackaged formulas that suggest they will are a ripoff.

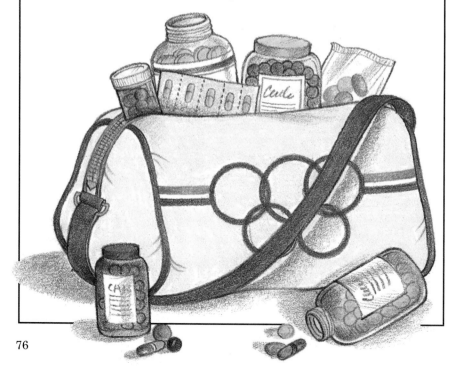

clear up a symptom, you should check with a doctor first.

NIACIN'S FLORID SIDE EFFECT

Guests at a New York brunch got a little something extra with their bagels recently, and it wasn't cream cheese.

Most of those who'd chosen the pumpernickel bagels found themselves blushing, flushing, itching and experiencing unpleasant heat in their skin. The bakers of this particular kind of bagel had confused niacin powder (used to fortify their dough) with a type of flour. Every bagel in that batch packed a niacin dose 15 times greater than the RDA.

But as the brunch guests soon found out from doctors, the "niacin flush" is short-lived and not dangerous. It is a common reaction to taking large doses of nicotinic acid, one form of niacin; up to 90 percent of those taking the vitamin experience it.

Do those who need a niacin supplement have to give it up? Not at all. Instead, they can simply switch to niacinamide, which is the same vitamin in a slightly different chemical package—one that doesn't cause the flush.

FLURRY OVER HERBS

Using herbs to treat disease generates controversy on two levels. The first level revolves around a discussion of whether they really work, or if their reputed healing effects are just so much nostalgic hokum and wishful thinking. The second level of controversy is whether they are safe to use—individually or in general.

The first argument is easy to settle. Herbs work. In fact, fully 25 percent of prescription drugs contain plant parts or chemical copies of them. Drugs based on herbs form the backbone of modern pharmaceuticals—including many of the anesthetics, as well as quinine, aspirin, morphine, the tranquilizer reserpine, the heart drug digitalis and several anticancer medications.

The second area of controversy, however, is not so easy to settle. Just like their modern chemical

---

Calcium Makes Bones, Not Stones

Almost everyone could benefit from taking extra calcium, the mineral that fights the brittle, porous, shrinking bones too often seen in the aging. But some people avoid supplements because they worry that calcium deposits will form in their joints, their heart or their kidneys.

Calcium takers need not worry. Even taking as much as 1,500 milligrams a day will have no effect on the tendency to form calcium deposits—a tendency that results from hormone imbalances or underlying damage to the tissues.

But you should know that some doctors believe you shouldn't take more than 2 grams of calcium a day, just to be on the safe side. For some individuals a larger amount might cause too high a level of the mineral in the blood. Marjorie Luckey, M.D., co-director of Mt. Sinai's Osteoporosis Clinic, believes that people who *do* have a tendency to form calcium deposits or kidney stones should be sure to take their mineral supplements under a doctor's supervision. They should also ask about the value of taking magnesium and vitamin B_6 for preventing kidney stones. Studies suggest that they work.

---

counterparts, herbs can have serious side effects. Some of these have come to light only recently as doctors searching for new medications took these time-honored plants into the lab for closer examination. However, to the dismay of many herbalists, some old favorites were unmasked as potential villains.

Unfortunately, not a lot of this information gets to the general public. Moreover, much of what does is frequently unreliable. Suppose you wanted to look up the herbs used in an old family remedy for coughs. If that remedy used coltsfoot, you'd probably be at a loss for solid information on which to base your decision. A book by an English physician says this herb is good for coughs. A second, this by a University of Utah professor, says, alarmingly, that "coltsfoot poisoning is unlikely." A third, by a pharmacologist, offers definitive proof that coltsfoot shouldn't be used at all because it may cause cancer.

Such is the case for many, many herbs. Available information is sketchy, confusing and frequently romanticized.

DANGER AHEAD

We do know that certain herbs—despite their undeniable mystique—are not considered safe to use. One such herb is comfrey.

When a popular health magazine recently published an article about the toxicity of comfrey, it was deluged with calls and letters from outraged comfrey fans who claimed the herb does everything except mind the children.

Those readers had reason to be nonplussed. Book after book tells just how wonderful comfrey is. But new evidence suggests that the plant causes liver cancer when fed to laboratory animals. An expert in drugs derived from plants, Ara Der Marderosian, Ph.D., of the Philadelphia College of Pharmacy and Science, says, "I would not recommend that comfrey tea be consumed at all, even in small doses."

Not all dangerous herbs are as familiar and old-fashioned as comfrey. People looking for the herbal equivalent of amphetamines have been victimized in recent years by a number of exotic offerings, like guarana, which contain caffeine as the primary stimulant.

Other mysterious, so-called pep pills contain worse. One writer felt like "a small-town mailbag snatched up by the express" after taking an alleged pep formula from a health food store. His heart raced, but his breathing almost outpaced it. The preparation he took was later shown to contain a potent prescription antiasthma drug.

Fortunately, some herbs do stand up to scientific scrutiny. One of them is garlic.

POTENT HERBS WITH POTENTIAL

Modern researchers are working with the odiferous plant and its oniony cousins to see if it truly does have therapeutic or preventative potential. What they've found is that garlic does indeed provide health benefits. It is a potent fighter of bacteria. In

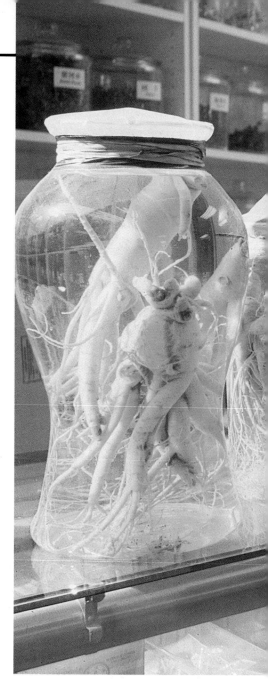

addition, it aids and abets digestion, fights atherosclerosis by reducing fats in the blood and even lowers high blood pressure. They've also found that the active ingredient does seem to be in the pungent part of the plant. So, as one scientist warns, the number of your acquaintances may be in an inverse ratio to the amount of your immunity.

THE FUTURE OF HERBS

A recent pharmaceutical convention chose as its symbol a crocus inside a benzene ring, suggesting a merger of the chemical with the natural. The symbol also reflects the increasing

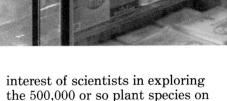

interest of scientists in exploring the 500,000 or so plant species on earth whose healing properties remain untested.

While scientists work, some laymen will continue herbal self-medication. For many, this treatment will be risky because of both the lack of regulation enforcing honest labeling and the abundance of misinformation about herbs in general. Anyone considering herbal treatments should, therefore, exercise extreme caution. Just like pharmaceutical drugs, herbs carry potential to harm rather than help your health. And like vitamin and mineral supplements, they should be swallowed with thought as well as with water.

Chinese Herbs

You may have noticed that Chinese herbs are turning up on health food store shelves, in fitness magazine ads and in your friends' conversation.

And you may have heard that Chinese herbology is based on over 2,000 years of healing experience and that more traditional Chinese doctors use herbs than use acupuncture. If your interest has been piqued, you might be considering trying some of these potions.

Unless you've studied Chinese medicine, however, self-prescribing Chinese herbs would be a little like a native Chinese going behind the counter of an American pharmacy and randomly selecting some miraculous Western medicines to take.

Second, what is commercially available as a Chinese herb may be neither an herb nor Chinese. Some so-called Chinese herbs have been found to contain toxic American prescription drugs.

A genuine Chinese herb treatment generally consists of 5 to 15 different compounds. And one of the things that makes it genuine is that each prescription is individual. So if you want Chinese herbs, seek out a traditional Chinese doctor.

Dangerous Herbs

Some herbs—camomile, peppermint, rosemary—are so pleasant that they become part of everyday living. Their aromatic comfort, however, may lead some people to believe that *all* herbs are benevolent, or at least benign.

Not so. What follows is a list of herbs that may cause trouble. You'll be surprised to find some old favorites on the list.

Herb	Description
Aconite	Call this herb wolfsbane. Ancient herbologists used this "queen mother of poisons" in deadly bait. Unsafe for wolves, human or otherwise.
Aloe	Fresh juice of the aloe plant helps heal minor wounds and burns. Scientists have verified it. But taken internally, it's a violent purge.
Angelica	Its sweet name contrasts with its devilish nature: It contains carcinogens. Women have been poisoned in futile attempts to induce abortion with it.
Apricot pits	The National Cancer Institute says the kernels and Laetrile made from them are totally useless to cancer patients. Worse, they contain cyanide.
Arnica	Using it internally "is folly," says one reliable text. It is toxic to the heart. It may be helpful when applied externally to bruises.
Bayberry bark	Is it useful as medicine? Not by any scientific measure, and rats get cancer when injected with it. The berries make nice candles, though.
Belladonna	A component of witch's brew, its name means beautiful lady. But its nicknames —deadly nightshade and dwale (for "trance")— are more apt. It's poisonous.
Bittersweet	Burning of the throat, nausea, vomiting, dizziness, lowered pulse and paralysis may be just the beginning. Just two berries can kill.
Bloodroot	Used by American Indians as a skin dye and to treat breast cancer, it shouldn't be used by reputable healers.
Blue cohosh	It cannot safely be used to stimulate menstruation or hasten childbirth, as some books suggest. It has a toxic effect on heart muscle and may hurt intestines.

Herb	Description
Broom	Although claimed by some to be a mood alterer when smoked, broom slows the heartbeat without making it stronger. It's a dangerous drug.
Calabar beans	In Africa, this herb was fed to suspected witches. If they lived, they were set free. Leave the berries of this highly toxic plant alone.
Calamus	Also known as sweet flag, this irislike flower has fallen into disrepute since animal studies showed it to cause heart and liver damage as well as cancer.
Camphor	This pungent stuff was once an ingredient of mothballs and may be useful in salves, but it's not healthy to ingest.
Celandine	Animals refuse to eat this, and people should, too. The sap from this poppylike plant causes severe stomach and intestinal irritation, and occasionally death.
Chaparral	Also called creosote bush and greasewood, it was on the FDA's "safe list" until 1970, when it was found to cause kidney and lymph node problems in rats.
Coltsfoot	If you want an herb for a cough, try slippery elm bark or marsh mallow root, not this herb that contains potent toxins that cause liver cancer.
Comfrey	"Definitely hazardous to health," one doctor of pharmacy calls it. This longtime favorite of herbalists has recently been shown to damage the liver.
Daffodils	If you're more inclined to gaze at them than eat them, you're on the right track. There is danger in munching the bulb.
Ergot	Actually a mold that grows on the rye plant, this stuff killed thousands in the Middle Ages. It's a base for potent drugs. Self-administration may be fatal.

Herb	Description	Herb	Description
Eyebright	Though the poet Milton had an angel clear Adam's sight with it, this flower that looks like bloodshot eyes may hurt yours, particularly if it's unsterilized.	**Mayflower**	Herbalists prescribed it to *lower* sexual excitement. And well it might with its nausea, colic, intestinal pain and kidney damage.
Foxglove	The source of the potent heart drug digitalis. An earlier use was as a "chemical jury"—if the accused took it and lived, he was innocent.	**Mistletoe**	Kiss under it, but don't kiss *it*. The berries and leaves may cause an agonizing disruption of the heartbeat and eventual death.
Gelsemium	Sometimes called yellow jasmine, it has been used as a painkiller, though other drugs are far more effective. It's not recommended for human consumption.	**Nux vomica**	The name alone should warn you off this one. It contains strychnine and is useful for poisoning moles.
Goldenseal	It makes you feel better—when you stop taking it. This extremely bitter herb makes some people nauseated. It has no effect below "near-toxic" doses.	**Pennyroyal**	"The herb has nothing to recommend it," says *The Honest Herbal*. One-half teaspoon of the oil caused convulsions and coma in one case.
Hellebore	Causes drooling, vomiting, falling heart rate and sudden drop in blood pressure. It's rarely fatal, though, because of the vomiting.	**Periwinkle**	A valuable source of modern drugs, it has been abused by the misguided seeking highs. It seriously depresses bone marrow function.
Henbane	Henbane is a poison. Thought by ancient peoples to have magical properties, this foul-smelling stuff causes delirium and a racing heartbeat.	**Pokeroot**	The word on this plant is "don't," and it should be written in neon. It has no known good effects. And children who've eaten the inky berries have died.
Jimsonweed	People have died trying to get high on this plant. Hallucinations may be paid for with an irregular heartbeat, elevated blood pressure and convulsions.	**Rue**	You'll rue the day you smell rue! So it may be effective as claimed as an insect repellent. It's also likely to cause a rash—on you. May upset stomach.
Juniper	It's not toxic in the tiny doses used to flavor gin (though you may think so next morning). But small, repeated doses may cause convulsions and kidney damage.	**Sassafras**	As little as a teaspon of the volatile oil causes degeneration of the heart, liver and kidneys. Do you really want that cup of tea?
Licorice	Don't worry about a licorice shoestring or two, but anyone with heart or blood pressure disorders should avoid this entirely.	**Spurge**	Another poisonous plant, this one has many names, but you don't want to swallow it no matter what it's called. The tea applied topically helps athlete's foot.
Life root	Its name reflects its old use, easing the pain of childbirth. Research reveals that it has little effect on the uterus, and worse yet, can damage the liver.	**Tansy**	"Should be used only with medical supervision," warns *Herbal Medications*, written by a doctor of pharmacy. Small quantities have caused death.
Lobelia	It's deadly. Sometimes sold as an aid to weight loss, it may work since "most individuals do not eat much when nauseated," says one book. It may be fatal.	**Tonka beans**	These atrophy the testicles of experimental animals. They retard growth, damage the liver and interfere with blood clotting.
Mandrake	Whether it's American mayapple or the European Satan's apple, mandrake is toxic. The European type destroys the heart and the American harms the intestines.	**Wormwood**	Once an ingredient in absinthe, it's a central nervous system depressant. Too much causes trembling, stupor, convulsions—and addiction.

6

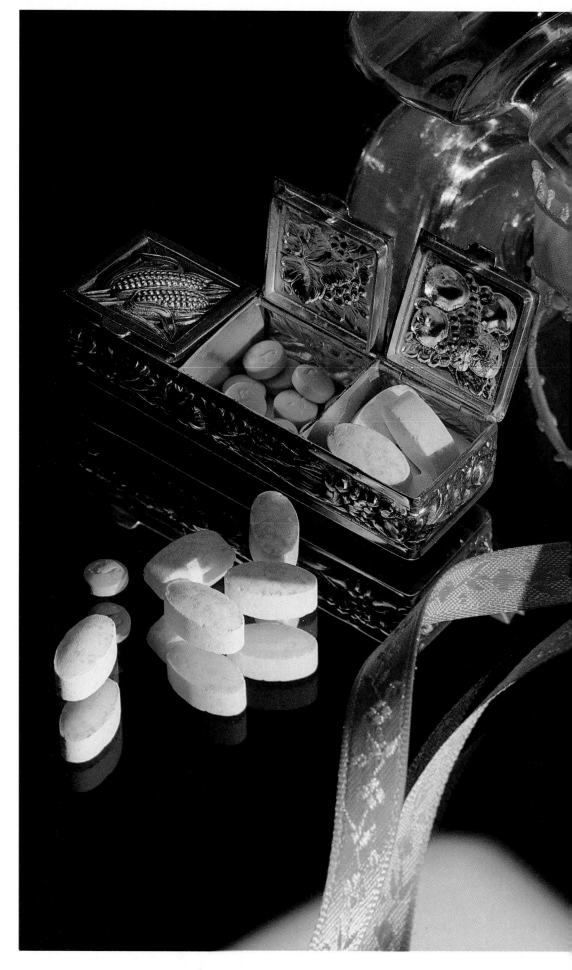

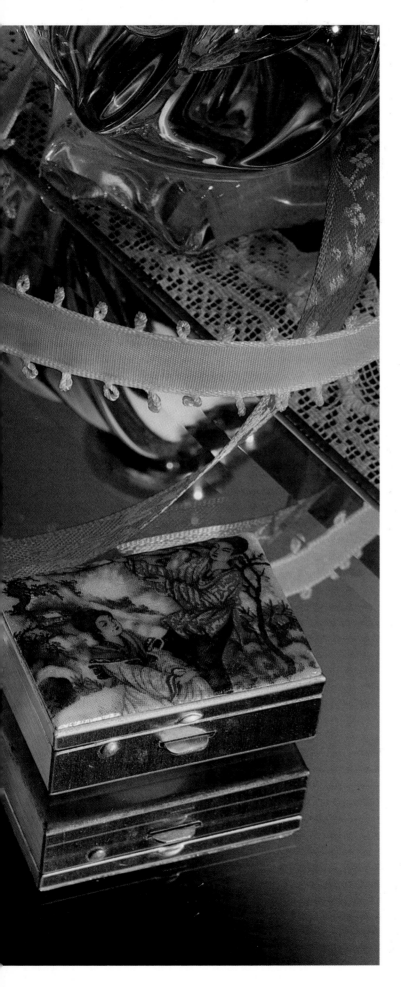

Women and Drugs

To be sure of getting
the best and safest drug or
contraceptive, learn about
the special needs of women.

E ven though more drugs are prescribed
for women than for men, doctors and other
health professionals may not know all they
should about the special way women respond to
certain medications.

Consider this very basic fact: Most men are
bigger than most women. Yet physicians can err
when they fail to note this difference in size. It's
unfortunate, but some doctors think of medications only in terms of what constitutes an "adult
dose." So, if a particular dosage of a drug is
correct for a 6-foot-tall man who weighs around
200 pounds, that same dosage would provide
almost twice as much drug per pound of body
weight for a woman who is just over 5 feet and
weighs 120 pounds.

The problem with that much extra medication in the bloodstream is that it can increase a
woman's chances of experiencing side effects from
too large a dose.

Differences in basic metabolism as well as in
the levels of circulating hormones also can make
women more susceptible to the side effects of
certain medications. Complicating the problem is
the fact that drug companies really don't know
how their drugs affect women, since most of their
testing is done on the male of the species (whether
that species be human or animal). This is done so
that researchers can avoid any effects caused by
the female hormonal cycle, which is often seen as
"a confounding variable in laboratory experiments,"
according to Jean Hamilton and Barbara Parry of
the National Institute of Mental Health. The
unfortunate result is that women report more
adverse drug reactions than men.

In addition to taking more medications in
general, women also take an additional group of
drugs developed specifically to help deal with
menstrual problems, contraception, fertility, menopause and associated areas where women display
special needs. Difficulties associated with
menstruation—cramps, crankiness and that bloated
feeling—are common to many women.

IS YOUR PERIOD A QUESTION MARK?

If it is, you're probably not satisfied with the medical advice you've been getting. "Don't get angry with the physicians," urges Ronald Norris, M.D. "Get mad at the people who trained them!"

Or, in some cases, at the people who didn't train them at all. Not only are medical schools stingy with lecture time devoted to the topic of menstruation and the female reproductive cycle, some even have reduced the study of obstetrics and gynecology to an elective subject.

This lack of knowledge only adds to the general confusion surrounding menstrual problems—and compounds the misunderstanding about one particular female complaint, premenstrual syndrome (PMS).

Although there is no uniformly accepted definition of PMS, M. Yusoff Dawood, M.D., professor of reproductive endocrinology at the University of Illinois College of Medicine in Chicago, has come up with what he calls a reasonable working definition: a clinical condition characterized by both physical and emotional symptoms that occur during the two weeks before menstruation and then disappear for at least a week after.

The most common of the hundred or more symptoms associated with PMS are the sadness, irritability and anxiety felt by 95 percent of the women with this condition.

Although doctors have responded to these symptoms in the past with a quick reach for the prescription pad, Dr. Norris, director of a PMS clinic in Massachusetts, cautions that drugs should be used sparingly. Tranquilizers, for example, serve as only a short-term measure in PMS.

When it comes to physical symptoms, Dr. Norris believes diuretics have been overprescribed. Although most women with PMS experience a feeling of being bloated, Dr. Norris points out that most, in fact, are not. They fail to show any weight gain, which means that fluid is not being retained, just redistributed throughout the body. He feels that the use of diuretics is appropriate only when a woman gains at least 3 pounds in the time just before her period.

If you are one of the few women who can honestly benefit from taking a diuretic, try to avoid the more powerful diuretics that can deplete the body's supply of potassium, which may cause muscle aches, cramps and—in very rare cases—death. Instead, ask your doctor to prescribe a mild potassium-sparing diuretic like Dyrenium.

HORMONE TREATMENTS

Another drug—one currently being used experimentally to treat PMS—not only works to eliminate the problem of fluid retention but also seems to alleviate mood symptoms. Called Spironolactone, it is a hormone which Dr. Norris calls the "drug of choice" for the problem. However, he points out that it's a steroid and therefore can have serious side effects.

Progesterone, also a hormone, has been used to treat more than 30,000 women in England over the last 30 years. Although critics contend there is no scientific proof that it works, others claim success rates of 90 percent. Dr. Norris is one of many who feel that progesterone is effective in treating a wide range of symptoms with minimal side effects and is especially effective against depression, anxiety and irritability.

Taking progesterone is not simple. It must be injected frequently into a fatty area, inserted as a vaginal suppository or applied rectally in liquid form. Since the vaginal and rectal preparations must be individually compounded, these products are expensive.

Oral contraceptives are yet another treatment for PMS, and one that Dr. Norris urges care in prescribing. In his experience, some women do improve with their use and some experience no effect at all, but *many* get much worse.

The good news is that more than half the women with PMS can control it without the use of drugs. They reduce or eliminate caffeine, salt, sugar and alcohol while eating more complex carbohydrates, whole

Wait for the Cramps

Some doctors tell women with painful periods to take nonsteroidal anti-inflammatory drugs (NSAIDs) a few days before their cramps actually begin, thereby preventing the buildup of prostaglandins, substances that may cause the discomfort.

Bad idea, counters reproductive endocrinologist M. Yusoff Dawood, M.D.

He points out that most women with the painful cramping of dysmenorrhea are young and sexually active and should avoid *any* drug whose effects on a possible undetected pregnancy are unknown.

Fortunately, ibuprofen and naproxen—two NSAIDs—are quick acting and effective when administered at the first sign of the menstrual flow.

---

grains and green leafy vegetables. They eat six small meals a day and get aerobic exercise. Some supplement their diet with vitamin B_6 and magnesium and try to limit stress.

UNCRAMPING YOUR STYLE

"If cramps are like a headache, then dysmenorrhea is a migraine," explains one sufferer. More than half of all women are affected by dysmenorrhea— painful periods—with some experiencing such severe pain that they are incapacitated for one to three days each month.

"Primary" dysmenorrhea usually occurs within a year of a young woman's first period and is linked to the period itself. "Secondary" dysmenorrhea is found in older women and is almost always a sign of a separate physical problem like endometriosis, fibroids or polyps.

It is important that women of any age see their doctor if they are experiencing pelvic pain, since endometriosis, a disease of the uterine lining, closely mimics dysmenorrhea.

Unfortunately, almost half the women with dysmenorrhea, even those with severe cases, do *not* consult a doctor and mostly use home remedies. What these women probably don't know is that there's one kind of medication that probably can banish their pain.

Known as nonsteroidal anti-inflammatory drugs (NSAIDs), they have been shown to provide relief in approximately 85 percent of women with dysmenorrhea.

Menstrual pain is caused by excessive uterine contractions that result from an overproduction of hormonelike chemical messengers known as prostaglandins. The NSAIDs work against the production of prostaglandins, thus removing the cause of the pain. Doctors recommend you continue to take them for the first three days of your period, even if the pain stops, to prevent the prostaglandins from building up.

Aspirin, the most common NSAID, is a weak prostaglandin inhibitor that most researchers agree is not effective for dysmenorrhea. Two prescription NSAIDs shown to be safe and effective are ibuprofen (Motrin) and naproxen (Anaprox).

Serious side effects have occurred with the use of some others, including indomethacin (Indocin). Reports indicate that almost half of all Indocin users experience side effects, including severe gastric irritation, headaches and a dizzy, spacey feeling. However, one-fourth of the people using Indocin have excellent results.

Dr. Dawood urges women to ask their doctors for the drug with the least side effects and the longest track record. He recommends Motrin as a first choice since it has been around the longest, works quickly and has few side effects. It's also the cheapest. Naproxen is his second choice.

CHOOSING A CONTRACEPTIVE

Although nine out of ten women of childbearing age use some form of birth control, contraception continues to be debated hotly from the laboratory to the pulpit. But for no one is the debate more personal than for the woman who does not want to become pregnant. Though technology has provided her with an astounding array of contraceptive methods, no one is ideal. Each day, some 33 million women choose what is, for them, the least of the evils.

The price of options is risk. Do you choose the method that kills 500 women a year or the one that kills only 30? In choosing conservatively, do you trade effectiveness for safety? An estimated 19,000 women are hospitalized each year for complications linked to use of the Pill and the IUD, two methods that are nearly foolproof. Few risks are associated with the use of the barrier methods, yet they are not as effective as more sophisticated contraceptives. Their main "risk" is getting pregnant—and more women die from the complications of pregnancy and childbirth than from the use of *any* birth control method.

While the choice is far from simple, the contraceptive risk can be calculated. A woman who has decided she does not want to become pregnant must take into account some of the same factors as the woman who wants to have a child: her age, income, lifestyle and medical history. To make a realistic choice, she has to know what's good and bad about each contraceptive method.

But using this delicate equation does not guarantee a perfect choice because it contains a blank, an "X" factor. The long-term effects of some methods, notably the Pill and the IUD, are still not known. It is not comforting to realize, as Judy Norsigian of the National Women's Health Network observes, that "we are all still guinea pigs in the contraception experiment."

But it can help when weighing risks known and unknown to put them in perspective. According to the Allan Guttmacher Institute, a research organization affiliated with Planned Parenthood, not only is it riskier to become pregnant than to use contraceptives, statistically speaking, it's also riskier to drive to the drugstore to have a prescription filled than to use any birth control method.

Every wise contraceptive decision is bolstered by good information, which in this case means realistic estimates of the health risks and benefits of each birth control method.

THE PILL

They are packaged for ultimate convenience: a small plastic case no larger than a purse mirror containing tiny pills arranged to be popped out one per day for either 21 or 28 days each month.

Easier to swallow than the average painkiller, the Pill is considerably more potent. At least 27 different compounds of various dosages are marketed in the United States, but most work in the same way: by suppressing ovulation. Normally, estrogen and progesterone are secreted at different phases of the monthly cycle to release a ripened egg from the ovary and to prepare the uterus to receive a fertilized egg. A pill containing synthetic estrogen and synthetic progesterone, which is called progestin, provides a constant level of hormones that tricks the regulating gland in the brain—the pituitary— into reacting as if a pregnancy has occurred. As a result, the ovary does not release a ripened egg, and conception can't take place.

As an added precaution, the progestin thickens the cervical mucus, which prevents the sperm from passing into the uterus. The Pill also has its own fail-safe system. It alters the uterine lining so that in the unlikely event an egg is produced and fertilized it can't implant itself in the womb.

To do this, the synthetic hormones in the Pill must be at least five times more powerful than those the body produces. Natural estrogen and progesterone are carried directly to the reproductive organs through the circulatory system. The synthetic versions take a roundabout route through the intestines and the liver, where the bulk of them is broken down.

THE GAMBLE

Needless to say, such a powerful drug causes dramatic changes in the

The Best Method for You

Method	Advantages	Disadvantages and Possible Side Effects	Who Shouldn't Use It
Pill	98 percent effective; convenient	Must be taken regularly. Common complaints include breast tenderness, nausea or vomiting, gain or loss of weight, breakthrough bleeding. Less common risks include blood clots, heart attack, stroke, high blood pressure, temporary post-Pill infertility, migraine headache, depression, gallbladder disease, liver tumors, diabetes.	Women who are over 35, smoke, are 20 pounds overweight, or who have any of the following disorders or a family history of them: high blood pressure, blood clots, high blood fats, heart disease, gallstones, diabetes, liver disorders, migraines, asthma, kidney disease, breast or uterine cancer.
Minipill	97 percent effective; may be safer because, compared to regular birth control pills, it contains very low levels of estrogen, which is linked to both the most life-threatening and minor side effects of Pill use.	Has a higher failure rate than combination pill; can cause irregular menses, decreased duration and amount of menstrual bleeding, breakthrough bleeding, amenorrhea.	Women who fit the profile given for the Pill. Also, women with breakthrough bleeding.
IUD	95 percent effective; once inserted, needs no further care except for periodic checks to make sure it is in place. Copper-coated IUDs must be changed every 3 years, the progesterone versions yearly.	May cause pain upon insertion, severe cramping and increased blood loss during menstruation; may be expelled; many hospitalizations are linked to IUD use. Other serious but rare side effects include anemia, pelvic inflammatory disease, uterine perforation, septic abortion, infertility.	Young women who eventually want to have children; women who are anemic, have cancer of the uterus or cervix, bleeding between periods or heavy flow, infection of any of the reproductive organs, venereal disease, severe cramps, copper allergy, abnormal Pap smear, any unexplained genital bleeding.
Diaphragm	87 percent effective; no discomfort or serious health risk such as those linked to Pill and IUD use; can be used by women who have infrequent intercourse; offers some protection against gynecological infections and sexually transmitted diseases.	Must be fitted by a physician and periodically refitted; requires a high level of motivation; can be inconvenient and messy to use; has a high failure rate because of incorrect use; can cause irritation; must be kept in for at least 6 to 8 hours after intercourse.	Women with "relaxed" vaginas or fallen uteruses.
Cervical cap	No recent studies on effectiveness—older studies show 85 to 99 percent; can be kept in place for days and weeks; frequent refitting isn't needed, as is often the case with diaphragms.	Can't be worn by women with irregularly shaped or slanted cervixes. Although a custom fitted version is now being tested, it's not approved by the FDA and is not readily available in the United States.	Women with irregularly shaped cervixes.
Condom	90 percent effective when used properly; easy to obtain and store; inexpensive; protects against venereal disease and infection.	Can reduce sexual sensation; may break or slip off during intercourse; interrupts sexual foreplay; can cause irritation, burning or an allergic reaction.	Couples who aren't highly motivated.
Spermicides	82 percent effective. Inexpensive; easy to obtain; no serious health risks except those linked to accidental pregnancy.	Must be used right before intercourse; effective for only about 30 minutes; messy; burning or irritation may occur; can cause allergic reaction.	No restrictions.
Contraceptive sponge	85 percent effective; easy to obtain and use; inexpensive; gives 24 hours of protection; one size fits all; needs no prescription or physician fitting.	Burning, irritation or allergic reactions may occur. Questions about potential carcinogenic properties and toxic shock syndrome linked to sponge use make it potentially hazardous.	No restrictions.

body right from the start. The ovaries, temporarily out of a job, shut down and begin to shrink. The uterus becomes softer and larger and takes on a bluish cast. The cervix also becomes soft and bluish. A woman taking oral contraceptives may also find her vagina is drier (even the pH changes) and she may become more susceptible to fungal infections.

But these may be the least of her worries. Oral contraceptive use is associated with a rogue's gallery of killer diseases, beginning with heart disease and stroke, which cause the majority of the 500 annual deaths linked to Pill use.

Age appears to be the Pill's chief partner in crime. The risk of heart attack and stroke for users under 25 is 4 per 100,000. For those between 25 and 34, the risk climbs to 13 per 100,000. But for Pill users over 35, the risk jumps to 54 per 100,000. In fact, 90 percent of all Pill-related risks are concentrated in the older age group, according to a

report by the Guttmacher Institute. High-estrogen pills carry the greatest health risk, and it is probably no coincidence that older Pill users, who skew the death statistics, are five times more likely to be taking a high-estrogen Pill.

In addition to age, smoking appears to be key to the dangers posed by oral contraceptives. A Pill user who smokes 25 or more cigarettes a day can increase her risk of heart attack by 20 to 40 times, according to a British study. The Guttmacher report estimates that the 500 deaths a year linked to Pill use could be reduced to a mere 70 if no Pill users smoked and no one took the Pill after age 35.

Pill users also run a high risk of high blood pressure and elevated blood fats (cholesterol and triglycerides), both significant factors in heart disease. They are also in greater danger of developing blood clots that can lead to stroke and pulmonary embolism, a clot in a major oxygen-carrying blood vessel. At blame is the estrogen in the Pill, which increases the production of a blood factor that promotes clotting.

Not only do Pill users find themselves at risk for a whole array of ailments, even their nutritional needs may change. Studies have shown that use of oral contraceptives can increase the body's requirements for riboflavin (vitamin B_2), vitamins B_6, B_{12} and C and folate and zinc.

And the dangers don't end when a woman stops taking the Pill. Some women experience menstrual irregularities, premenstrual problems and severe cramps after they go off oral contraceptives, which, ironically, are often prescribed to alleviate those conditions. A study also indicated that nearly a quarter of the women who go off the Pill may be unable to conceive for more than a year. However, this post-Pill infertility seems to be temporary. Some doctors also recommend that women not attempt to conceive in the first few cycles after stopping the Pill because of the increased risk of miscarriage and birth defects.

Though the Pill may sound as harmless as the neutron bomb, it should be remembered that the major-

Some Drugs Can Undo Your Contraceptive

If you are taking antibiotics for an infection and a low-estrogen Pill for contraception, you could be increasing your risk of an unwanted pregnancy. Some antibiotics may alter the way the body breaks down estrogen. There may be increased excretion of the hormone in the feces, resulting in a reduced blood concentration and a corresponding reduction in the effectiveness of your Pill.

Several other drugs are known to compromise the efficacy of oral contraceptives. They include the antibiotic rifampin; the tranquilizers Miltown and Equanil; Butazolidin, a drug used in the treatment of arthritis and joint injuries; barbiturates such as sleeping pills; and the anti-seizure drugs Dilantin, phenobarbitol, primidone and ethosuximide.

Women who take these drugs as well as oral contraceptives may have to adjust their Pill dosage or take added precautions—use of the barrier methods, for instance—for as long as they use the medication.

ity of Pill users experience only minor side effects if any, and many of these can be eliminated by changing Pills or dosage.

THE IUD

Legend has it that the first IUDs were pebbles inserted by Arab camel drivers into the uteruses of their animals to prevent inconvenient pregnancies on the long treks across the desert. But ancient as this birth control device may be, no one is really sure how it works.

But work it does: It is the most effective contraceptive after the Pill. But for many women, it is also one of the most frightening. Although it has one of the lowest death rates among all contraceptive methods, there are significantly more hospitalizations resulting from IUD use. Nine out of ten are for treatment of pelvic inflammatory disease (PID), a serious, often virulent infection of the reproductive organs that is a major cause of infertility. It is not clear why the IUD increases a woman's risk of PID. Some experimental evidence suggests that the IUD's nylon tail—which hangs into the cervix to make it easier to tell if the device is still in place—may be the avenue by which vaginal bacteria creep up into the uterus.

PID risk is lowest among users of copper-coated IUDs and highest among women who use a controversial device called the Dalkon Shield. The makers of this IUD, A.H. Robins Company, voluntarily withdrew it from the market after 36 reported cases of septic (infected) pregnancies, 4 of which resulted in death.

Another serious, if rare, side effect is uterine perforation. Of the 875 cases that occur yearly, most happen during or just after insertion and are linked not to the device itself but to the skill of the health professional who inserts it. For these reasons, women who use the Dalkon Shield are being urged by both the manufacturers and health-care professionals to have it removed.

Although IUD users have a lower-than-average risk of tubal pregnancy, an IUD user who does become pregnant is more likely to

have a spontaneous abortion.

But the majority of women who eventually give up the IUD do so not because of these severe but rare side effects, but because of expulsion, severe cramping and heavy menstrual bleeding and spotting. With an IUD, menstrual blood loss can double or triple and some women have periods lasting nearly two weeks. Recent studies have shown that one device— the Copper 7, which is the smallest and the one most often used by women who have not had children—is responsible for the most between-period spotting and the longest duration of menstrual bleeding. Ironically, it does not produce the largest blood loss. That honor goes to the Lippes Loop, according to researchers in Oxford, England.

Nonetheless, the IUD is the fourth most popular contraceptive in the United States. It's also one of

---

Contraception: What the Future Holds

When the new century dawns, don't expect to see many revolutionary changes in contraception. What scientists foresee are simply variations on a theme:

Injectables like Depo-Provera give 3 months of protection with a single shot of progestin.

Subdermal implants like Norplant, developed by The Population Council, are tiny rods containing 35 milligrams of the progestin levonorgestrel that are placed in the upper arm and offer 5 years of highly effective protection.

Unisex contraceptives may debut. A synthetic brain hormone, administered via a nasal spray, has been shown to inhibit ovulation in women and the production of sperm in men.

Gossypol, a derivative of the cotton plant, has been shown in Chinese studies to inhibit the production of sperm.

The vaginal ring, smaller than the rim of the diaphragm, slowly releases a progestational agent that thickens cervical mucus to prevent sperm from passing into the uterus. It has to be worn continuously.

Period prompters start menstruation even if fertilization has occurred, sweeping out the implanted ovum with the uterine lining.

the more expensive, costing about $131 in the first year.

THE BARRIER METHODS

The barrier methods—the diaphragm, cervical cap, condom, sponge and spermicides—are so called because they either block the passage of sperm into the cervix or kill those that slip through. Because of bad publicity surrounding the Pill and IUD, these fairly risk-free methods are enjoying renewed popularity.

Another reason for their popularity may be that they are among the least expensive forms of birth control on the market today. Condoms, spermicides and the contraceptive sponge are all available without prescription.

The condom is probably the oldest contraceptive, invented in the 16th century to prevent syphilis. Made from rubber or lamb membrane, this small sheath fits snugly over the penis and catches ejaculated semen. Condoms can be the most effective of the barrier methods, about 90 percent effective when used alone and an astounding 98 to 99 percent effective when used with a spermicide.

But they can't work if they aren't used, or are used improperly—the chief reasons for the contraceptive failure of the condom.

DIAPHRAGMS AND CAPS

The diaphragm is a cap-shaped cup made of rubber. It covers the cervix to prevent sperm from swimming into the uterus. There are three common types, all with spring-fitted rims that can be compressed for easy insertion and that "spring" back to fit snugly against the vaginal wall and cervix. Used in tandem with spermicide and a hefty dose of motivation, a diaphragm can be nearly as effective as an IUD. Unfortunately, the actual failure rate is significantly higher than that of either the Pill or the IUD.

Many things can go wrong. The diaphragm, which must be fitted by a doctor and purchased by prescription, can be sized incorrectly or inserted improperly. It can be jostled loose during intercourse or not used because it interferes with the spontaneity of the romantic moment. Some women find it annoying and remove it after intercourse, although it must be kept in place for at least 6 to 8 hours to ensure that all the sperm are dead. It also is the second most expensive method, costing about $160 in the first year if obtained from a private physician.

Similar to the diaphragm in looks and effectiveness is the cervical cap. The small, thimble-shaped device fits over the cervix, where it is held in place by suction that creates an airtight seal. The diaphragm, on the other hand, covers the cervix and surrounding area and is held in place by tension against the vaginal walls. Both are used with spermicide.

The cap's advantage over the diaphragm is that it can be inserted hours or days before intercourse and can be kept in for hours or days afterwards. But it must be removed during menstruation to allow the release of menstrual fluids.

SPERMICIDES AND SPONGES

The active ingredient in spermicides is a detergent that kills sperm by creating a hostile environment in the vagina. And spermicides are the active component of the contracep-

Vitamin C for Fertility

The fertility drug Clomid has a good success rate—but it's not perfect. Masao Igarashi, M.D., a Japanese gynecologist, tried to improve the effectiveness of Clomid by adding vitamin C to the treatment regimen, and even attempted to induce fertility by using vitamin C alone. The results?

In 2 out of 5 women who habitually failed to ovulate and who hadn't responded to Clomid therapy, vitamin C alone caused ovulation. In 5 other cases, vitamin C and Clomid combined corrected the problem. (Use vitamin C for this problem only under the supervision of your doctor.)

tive sponge, a powder-puff-like device made of polyurethane that has been available since 1983.

Spermicides come in creams, jellies, foams and suppositories, but the most effective are the foams that are placed deep in the vagina and spread across the cervix during intercourse. Spermicide protection is generally short-lived: only 30 minutes. But the sponge contains about 24 hours worth of protection, so it can be inserted almost any time before intercourse.

Effectiveness rates can be high—higher than for the condom—but the failure rates are high, too. The spermicides are most effective when used with another method, the condom or diaphragm, for instance. There seem to be no serious health risks, outside of accidental pregnancy, associated with the spermicides. In fact, there are actually some health benefits. Recent studies have shown that spermicide users have a low rate of gonorrhea and may be less likely to get herpes.

The sponge is moderately effective, with a failure rate of about 15 to 16 percent, but it is remarkably convenient. It's one-size-fits-all, needs no physician fitting and can be left in place for repeated intercourse.

It's the favorite method of about a half million women, but it has already fallen out of favor with many birth control experts because of questions about the possible carcinogenic properties of the sponge and the spermicides it contains and several reported cases of toxic shock syndrome (TSS) associated with its use. Some health professionals are also concerned that the sponge may encourage some infections by blocking the natural cervical secretions.

DRUGS FOR INFERTILITY

For most people, it's the most natural thing in the world. Natural, but a miracle—one that happens when a couple expresses their love.

For 14 percent of all American couples—5 million people—the miracle, unfortunately, has been replaced with misery and heartbreak. The problem is infertility, and it's on the rise.

Cure a Cough, Have a Baby

Take some cough syrup and go to bed. While it sounds like a cure for a cold, it's really a suggestion for treating infertility, according to a Philadelphia obstetrician, Jerome Check, M.D. To treat 40 women whose cervical mucus was unable to transport sperm, he administered guaifenesin, an active ingredient in some OTC cough remedies. Twenty-three showed marked improvement in the quality of their cervical mucus, and 16 eventually became pregnant. Seems this drug can thin out mucus anywhere in the body, without the side effects of other therapies. If you want to try it, call your doctor for details.

Fortunately, infertility usually can be reversed. "Once there wasn't much you could do about it beyond bowing to the local fertility gods. Today, there are many things we can do about infertility, starting with accurate diagnosis and ending with effective treatment, just like any other medical condition," says William Andrews, M.D., professor of obstetrics and gynecology at the Eastern Virginia Medical School in Norfolk.

But what *kind* of treatment? It appears that women are automatically put on drugs that make them produce a litter of offspring. But appearances can be deceptive. Not all fertility drugs boost a woman's hormones into overdrive and make her ovulate wildly. The term fertility drugs represents a wide range of medications, each with very different effects, each prescribed for a specific condition.

ANOVULATORY DRUGS: HORMONAL OVERDRIVE

It's only when a woman isn't ovulating that doctors prescribe a drug that might result in multiple births. The drug of choice for anovulatory infertility—the one least likely to produce more than one baby—is serophene, or Clomid, because of its low cost and safety. It fools the body into thinking that estrogen levels are lower than they really are, setting off the hormones that induce ovulation. As many as 80 percent of the women put on this drug ovulate, with half becoming pregnant.

Parlodel is newer than Clomid and more spectacularly successful. One study boasted a pregnancy rate of 96 percent, better than for any other course of treatment. Its principal use, however, is to treat infertility caused by too-high levels of the hormone prolactin, a relatively rare condition. Prolactin stimulates milk flow and breast growth, but if there's

Are Your Drugs Rated X?

When it becomes necessary to take medication for a serious problem during pregnancy, how can you (and your doctor) determine which antibiotic, for example, may be safer than others? The FDA has instituted a simple safety-during-pregnancy code that you can look up in the *Physicians' Desk Reference (PDR)* to give you some guidance. Lloyd Millstein, Ph.D., director of the FDA's division of drug advertising and labeling, explains the categories:

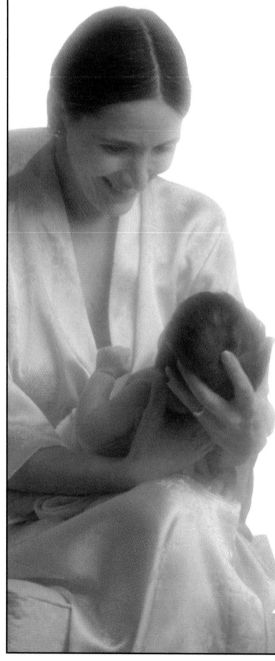

A—Drugs are given grade A when available evidence indicates that their benefits greatly outweigh the risks. This includes drugs (like thyroid medications) that may not be absolutely safe but are *necessary* for the mother's health.

B—As with all drugs, there is still some risk, but the FDA labels B only those drugs that appear reasonably safe after extensive animal tests and follow-up studies on women who took the drug while pregnant and reported any effects on them or their babies.

C—Since more risk is thought to be involved, physicians are urged to look for safer alternatives, especially in the first trimester. Ideally, these drugs should be reserved for special cases—if the woman is allergic to safer drugs or there is a lack of safer drugs.

D—Look hard for safer alternatives. Drugs in this category pose a very strong risk of serious harm to the fetus. Also labeled D are drugs a pregnant woman can do without (like Valium).

X—This letter was chosen to stand out. It means *doctor be careful; patient beware!* The risks involved outweigh any possible benefit from the drug, as documented by numerous reports. The acne medication Accutane falls into this category.

Dr. Millstein explains that C is a "normal" grade. Drug companies must provide proof of safety to get a B, while some evidence of danger is needed to give a drug a D. When grading the drugs, the FDA also takes into account *why* a drug would be taken.

too much of it, it inhibits the hormone progesterone, which is essential for ovulation.

And Parlodel has a very high rate of side effects—up to 68 percent of all women taking the drug experience dizziness, drowsiness, lightheadedness, nausea or headaches. For many women, though, the desire for a baby may outweigh the problem of side effects.

The ultimate treatment for failure to ovulate is Pergonal. Used only when no other drug works, its potential side effects—multiple births, enlargement of the ovaries—are serious.

Distilled from the urine of postmenopausal women, Pergonal acts by hyperstimulating two hormones called FSH and LH, which in turn help to stimulate ovulation.

In the past, the result may have been quintuplets, but with daily estrogen monitoring to see how much Pergonal is needed, the risk of multiple births has been reduced to less than 20 percent.

Technology hasn't done anything to improve Pergonal's two main disadvantages, however: the way it's used and its cost. Pergonal must be injected, and a cycle of treatments can cost up to $3,000.

CAUTIONS AND HOPE

Fertility counselors urge women taking any fertility drug to do some monitoring of their own. "We recommend they are aware of potential side effects, and we strongly encourage patients taking these drugs to work very closely with their doctors and challenge them when necessary. It's a collaborative effort. You don't just turn control of your body over to your physician."

In some cases infertility is not treated with drugs at all. In fact, many times the condition is corrected with surgery—opening blocked fallopian tubes, removing cysts, correcting uterine or vaginal abnormalities or eliminating endometriosis. And in 40 percent of all couples who are infertile the woman isn't treated at all—her husband is.

And if none of these treatments work, there's still hope. A study of over 1,000 infertile couples found that 61 percent of those who had a child did so from 2 to 6½ years *after* treatment had been stopped. Ultimately, nature just took its course. "We conclude that the potential for a spontaneous cure for infertility is high," the report concluded.

DRUGS IN PREGNANCY—THE FEWEST AND THE SAFEST

While doctors agree that a drug-free pregnancy is ideal and that today's woman is taking fewer drugs during pregnancy, they also recognize that around 90 percent of all pregnant women will still take some drugs.

Some will take medications to ease problems caused by the pregnancy itself, like morning sickness. Others either enter the pregnancy with a serious physical problem or develop one during it. And for all mothers-to-be there are the choices to be made about drugs during labor and delivery.

The mother-to-be is faced with a lot of decisions. Should she take a medicine she needs with little regard for its effects on her unborn child, or should she tough-out an illness—protecting her baby but possibly harming herself?

The answer lies somewhere in between. The FDA cautions pregnant women to use drugs *only when necessary.* Doctors agree, adding that women who have a real medical problem should not try to do without medication, but should try to find the safest drug available. Improving your own health can improve that of the fetus as well, they say.

COLDS, NO; INFECTIONS, YES

"I don't like my patients taking an antihistamine for a cold even when they're *not* pregnant," says Robert Brent, M.D., professor and chairman of the department of pediatrics at Thomas Jefferson University Hospital in Philadelphia. Experts agree that no medicine can cure a cold and that nonmedical treatments often can replace drugs to relieve symptoms.

Dr. Brent points out that over-the-counter drugs should be evaluated just as carefully as their prescription counterparts. He warns women to especially avoid cold preparations that contain iodide, which he says may harm the developing thyroid of the fetus.

While bed rest and lots of liquids may be the way to handle a cold, infections such as pneumonia require medical treatment. Dr. Brent says, "If an antibiotic is justified, it has to be used," even during pregnancy.

One antibiotic, tetracycline, is well known for its potential side effect of staining the teeth developing in the fetus and slowing its bone growth. What isn't well known is that this antibiotic also can affect the mother directly by damaging her liver.

Luckily, safe alternatives are available and mothers in need are cautioned not to reject antibiotics out of hand. Rather, they should work with their doctors to choose the safest treatment for their problem.

WHEN DRUGS AND PREGNANCY MIX

It is estimated that one in every five women begins pregnancy with a previously existing medical disorder. For those with serious problems like hypertension, diabetes, blood clots, thyroid disorders, epilepsy or cancer, experts agree that medication not only is justified but that in some cases it's the only way these women can have a successful pregnancy.

"Fifty years ago a diabetic woman couldn't hope to have a child," says Dr. Brent, pointing out that better medicine has increased the chances of such "high-risk" women becoming pregnant.

But despite their high-risk designation, these women still have excellent chances for a successful outcome. Drugs taken during pregnancy are thought to account for no more than 5 percent of all birth defects, while a mother with chronic high blood pressure faces the awful statistic of a fetal death rate of up to 40 percent if she attempts her pregnancy without the aid of carefully chosen medications.

CHANGE OF LIFE

As surely as every female passes into the age of childbearing, so she will go through another change—usually between the ages of 48 and 52—that turns off the process.

The reproductive stage of life stops because the ovaries and other tissues decrease the production of the hormone estrogen. Unfortunately, after 35-odd years of keeping the female body moving to its own special rhythm, estrogen doesn't just stop overnight. Instead, estrogen levels become erratic—fluctuating sometimes for months or even years, depending on the individual. These cause some unpleasant times for many women going through "the change." And hot flashes, dry vagina and the prospect of bone loss head the list of the most common symptoms of menopause.

For more than 20 years the popular method of treatment has been this: Simply replace the diminishing amount of estrogen (the cause of all the discomfort) with a synthetic form of estrogen and the symptoms (for the most part) vanish.

THE PROGESTIN CONNECTION

Estrogen Replacement Therapy, or ERT as it is known, is not without its share of controversy. For one thing, it carries with it an element of risk—namely an increased chance of developing uterine (endometrial) cancer, in addition to other woes (see "Commonsense Guide to Estrogen Replacement Therapy"). However, these risks may have been reduced somewhat over the last several years with the addition of progestin—the synthetic form of progesterone—to the treatment process. Progestin protects the lining of the uterus from the damaging effects of the estrogen. In fact, there is reason to believe that it may even provide some protection *against* cancer. (The jury isn't in on progestin, however. Some researchers believe that it, too, may carry the same risks as taking *any* hormone and they urge caution.) Also reducing the risks of ERT, estrogen is now given in smaller doses than it was during the 1970s.

Commonsense Guide to Estrogen Replacement Therapy

Types of Treatment	Rationale for Prescribing	Possible Drawbacks	Possible Benefits	Ways to Minimize Risks	Alternatives
Estrogen alone (Premarin, Menest, Estratabs and Evex are common drug names)	Replacement of estrogen; prevention or alleviation of hot flashes, dry vagina and problems such as painful urination and incontinence; prevention of brittle bones caused by demineralization and loss of calcium; treatment of osteoporosis	Continuation of menstrual flow; postmenopausal uterine bleeding; stroke; high blood pressure; cancer of uterus; breast cancer; gallbladder disease; fibroid tumors; possible dependency	Prevention of bone loss; protection against heart disease; decreased levels of LDL (bad) cholesterol; increased levels of HDL (good) cholesterol	Take lowest possible dose for shortest possible time; supplement diet with adequate amounts of vitamins B_1, B_2, B_6, C, E and folate and zinc; check out vaginal bleeding immediately with physician; wean gradually from estrogen to adjust body to diminishing amounts	Vitamins E and C; bioflavonoids; icy beverages; stress management; calcium, vitamin D and exercise
Progestin alone (Depo-Provera, Norlutate are common drug names)	Relief of hot flashes when a woman's state of health prohibits estrogen use; some protection against thinning bones	Greater risk of vaginal dryness; irregular vaginal bleeding; mild, temporary depression; weight gain; possible irregular menstrual cycles; must be injected; is used as effective contraceptive in some countries but has not been approved by FDA in U.S. because it has caused cancer in lab animals	Elimination of flashes and sweats	*See* Estrogen alone	*See* Estrogen alone
Estrogen and progestin	*See* Estrogen alone	*See* Estrogen alone. The addition of progestin may reduce the possible health risks; its long-term effects may be harmful, however.	*See* Estrogen alone. Acts much like birth control pills but dosage is not strong enough to protect against conception; carries no greater risk of blood clots than taking no drug at all.	*See* Estrogen alone	*See* Estrogen alone
Topical estrogen creams (Premarin, Ogen, DV, Estraguard are common drug names)	Relief of pain during sexual intercourse due to drying and thinning of vaginal wall; reduction of minor difficulty in urinating.	Absorption of estrogen in bloodstream; possible bleeding after menopause	Relief of vaginal soreness and pain during sex; help in prevention of vaginal discharge	Use sparingly and only according to doctor's directions; not safe for women with breast cancer	K-Y lubricating jelly; vegetable oils

Estrogen? Progestin? Sound a little like a birth control formula to you? Well, it is. In fact, both birth control and ERT are taken in a similar fashion. But there is a noticeable difference between the two. The quantity of hormones used in ERT is a lot less than that in oral contraceptives, meaning ERT cannot be considered protection against pregnancy. Because the dosage is much lower, ERT does not carry the same health risks as birth control pills. In fact, the risk of blood clots—a major concern with oral contraceptives—is no higher for women having ERT than for those who take no drugs at all.

HOW THE TREATMENT WORKS

If you've ever taken birth control pills, you're already familiar with the treatment schedule—three weeks on the hormones followed by one week off. Prior to starting ERT, a thorough breast and pelvic examination, including a Pap smear, is mandatory.

The most commonly prescribed ERT contains a mixture of several synthetic estrogens. Premarin is the most popular combination.

Estrogen should always be given at the lowest possible dose and from days 1 to 25 of the treatment cycle. Oral progestin should be added on days 16 to 25. (Since the progestin is added to protect the uterus, it obviously is not necessary for those who have had a hysterectomy.) Dosage should be increased only if the symptoms are not relieved after a one-month cycle of therapy.

Women with heart disease, high blood pressure, diabetes, migraine headaches or large uterine fibroids should never consider ERT.

WHO NEEDS ERT?

ERT should not be entered into lightly. For one thing, while hot flashes and a dry vagina are a very real and very discomforting part of menopause, few women have symptoms severe enough to warrant such drastic treatment. And while estrogen can be helpful in preventing the bone-loss disease known as osteoporosis, some doctors feel that supplemental calcium and vitamin D—alone or in combination with estrogen—can be used to prevent it. As for painful intercourse due to dry vagina, lubricants like K-Y jelly or even estrogen creams (you'll still be getting the hormone into your system, but not as much) work quite nicely.

Just remember, even though the risks of ERT to your health may have been diminished, the risks get greater the longer you stay on the treatment. So it's wise to elect how you'll handle your time of menopause just as you would elective surgery—with careful consideration and consultation with a trusted doctor.

DISEASES THAT COME FROM INTIMACY

An expression favored during the turbulent 1960s was, "If you're not part of the solution, you're part of the problem." Today that especially holds true for people with sexually transmitted diseases (STDs). If you have a venereal disease, you can solve the problem with a cure or become part of it by not treating the disease and therefore spreading it to others.

Failure to obtain proper treatment for yourself and your partner can have devastating consequences, since symptoms of venereal disease may disappear while the disease itself continues to flourish.

STDs include such well-known problems as syphilis, gonorrhea and herpes, as well as lesser-known but extremely common conditions like chlamydia and pelvic inflammatory disease. These infections are caused by bacteria, viruses, fungi and protozoa. When correctly administered, antibiotics can cure all the STDs except herpes—and there's even a drug to help with that disease's painful symptoms.

The most effective drug used to fight STDs is penicillin, explains Yehudi Felman, M.D., director of New York City's bureau of VD control. The potential dangers are limited to those who are allergic to it.

Most people who are penicillin sensitive will develop only itchy, elevated patches on the skin. Less common—but life-threatening when untreated—are shock and difficulty in breathing. If you're not sure whether you're allergic to penicillin, you can be tested. Dr. Felman feels that the problem of penicillin sensitivity is not serious; with so many good alternatives to the drug available, he simply uses something else.

DANGEROUS BUT CURABLE

Called "the great impostor" because its symptoms mimic those of many other diseases, syphilis is dangerous but curable. Cases detected early are usually treated with a single massive dose of penicillin G benzanthine. More advanced syphilis requires similar injections weekly.

What happens if you're allergic to penicillin? In less advanced cases, a person is advised to take oral tetracycline for up to 30 days. Those who can't tolerate tetracycline can use erythromycin, which is also the drug of choice for pregnant women.

THREE MILLION VICTIMS

For the three million unfortunates who will contract gonorrhea this year, the treatment is a massive injection of another form of penicillin (called aqueous pencillin G procaine) into two sites in one visit. The injections are accompanied by a pill called probenecid. This so-called helper drug keeps penicillin in the body so that it has longer to do its work. This treatment also gets rid of incubating syphilis, if you're unfortunate enough to have both.

Certain "resistant" strains of gonorrhea are not killed by penicillin. In fact, they actually produce an enzyme that attacks the drug. But Dr. Felman says that these resistant strains account for, at most, 2 percent of the gonorrhea in the U.S., although it can be as high as 50 percent in other parts of the world. The antibiotic spectinomycin works well in those cases.

If you are allergic to penicillin, one alternative is to take oral tetracycline. This treatment can be difficult because you have to take four pills a day at different times for a week; you have to take them at least an hour before or 2 hours after meals; and you must avoid dairy products. Doctors agree that this schedule is difficult to follow correctly and that some people fail to cure their problem because they don't finish up all the pills or take them at the wrong times.

Fortunately, a newer drug, doxycycline, is just as effective and you need only two pills a day. Cost, however, can be a problem. Dr. Felman points out that doxycycline is ten times more expensive than tetracycline.

PELVIC INFLAMMATION

Pelvic inflammatory disease, an infection of the uterus and fallopian tubes that can spread to other areas and lead to sterility, is a serious health problem for women. The CDC points out that many experts recommend that *all* PID patients be hospitalized so that treatment can be closely monitored.

There are no absolutes when it comes to fighting the diverse organisms that cause the infection, and women with the problem will be treated with combinations of antibiotics that are effective against a large number of the little nasties. Treatment begins with intravenous administration of the drugs until two days after the accompanying fever breaks, and then continues with oral antibiotics to complete two weeks of therapy.

HERPES RELIEF

Everyone knows that diamonds and herpes are forever. Even though there's no cure for the latter, an ointment called acyclovir can help reduce the pain and speed the healing *of the first outbreak only.* Wearing gloves, you spread it over the lesions three times a day for one week. It doesn't prevent recurrences and it has not yet been tested for safety during pregnancy.

One drug that's definitely not safe during pregnancy is podophyllin, a solution that's painted on venereal warts. Dr. Felman warns of its extreme toxicity, which can poison your system if used on too large an area or if not washed off quickly enough.

(continued on page 100)

Not for Women Only

If you have one of the STDs, your sex partners may have it as well. They may feel fine. They may have no symptoms at all. They will *still* reinfect you. All the experts agree: You *must* contact your contacts and each of you must be treated at the same time to avoid passing the problem back and forth. Remember, they may show no symptoms, but what they don't see is what you *will* get.

The Feminine Hygiene Myth

Looking at advertisements for feminine hygiene products, you'd think women really were searching for what author Carol Ann Rinzler calls "a plastic vagina, nice and clean and totally devoid of human scent."

Ms. Rinzler, author of *Strictly Female, an Evaluation of Brand-Name Health and Hygiene Products for Women* says that because women fear both odor and uncleanliness, millions of them buy feminine hygiene products to help them cure a "problem" that really isn't a problem at all.

The healthy vagina is at once an efficient yet complex body system that under normal circumstances maintains itself. It washes itself out, it harbors good microorganisms that keep it healthy and it prevents the bad organisms from multiplying out of control.

Products that allegedly keep the vagina cleaner and/or fresher-smelling may do more to harm its self-maintaining system than they do to help it. Here's a rundown on the most common products.

Douches

To understand how douches may upset the vagina's natural defense system, let's look first at how the system works. Perhaps the most important protective system is the acid balance. A healthy vagina is usually slightly acidic. Acidity prevents many different kinds of bothersome bacteria and other microorganisms from flourishing.

A second protective system is the cervical mucus. Although some women think of the mucus as unclean, just the opposite is true. Normal discharge (which is odorless and fluctuates between a clear egg-white consistency and a milky white paste) bathes the vaginal walls, washing away dead cells and other debris. It also lubricates the vaginal walls to protect them from damage and plugs the cervical opening to defend the uterus from the invasion of unfriendly bacteria and other microorganisms.

A lot of factors can contribute to upsetting the vagina's protective systems. Stress, anxiety and lack of sleep can upset the acid balance. So can other conditions, such as pregnancy or menstruation. Antibiotics also can make you more prone to infections.

With all of these hard-to-control factors (who can avoid stress or menstruation?), why, then, do women add to their vulnerability by douching?

Here's how douching can throw your vaginal system off-kilter in a number of ways.

Douching dries out the cervical mucus so essential to a healthy vagina. This lack of mucus can cause irritation or damage to the vaginal walls. It can also upset your acid balance, further setting you up for infections.

Done improperly, douching can actually propel microorganisms from the vagina into the uterus. It's a particularly bad idea to douche during menstruation or pregnancy or when the cervix is dilated and the upward flow can bring infected material into the uterus.

"Most gynecologists do not recommend the practice of douching, primarily because it doesn't do much good and can cause trouble," say William F. Rayburn, M.D., Frederick P. Zuspan, M.D., and Jeanne T. Fitzgerald, authors of *Every Woman's Pharmacy*.

If you're douching to clear up a case of vaginitis (the catch-all term for inflammations of the vagina), you'd be better off trying a sitz bath instead. Add ½ cup of salt or white vinegar to warm, shallow bath water, sit in the tub with your feet propped up on either side, and insert a finger into the vagina to help the solution enter.

Feminine Hygiene Sprays

While some may see a health rationale for trying a douche (the belief that it "cleans out" the vagina), no such excuse exists for feminine hygiene sprays. These products come under the heading of cosmetics, not medications. Their primary ingredient is perfume and their sole purpose is to mask so-called odors in the female genital region.

Because of their perfume content, feminine hygiene sprays can cause irritation and inflammation of the delicate tissues in the vulva and vagina. They also can cause allergic reactions. Besides, according to *Every Woman's Pharmacy*, most evidence indicates that washing daily achieves the same deodorizing effect as the sprays—without the side effects.

Premoistened Towelettes

Like feminine hygiene sprays, premoistened towelettes are a product with no reason for being. In fact, they can leave your vaginal area too moist, which makes it a perfect breeding ground for unfriendly bacteria and other irritation-causing organisms, according to Ms. Rinzler. On top of that, premoistened towelettes contain the same irritating perfumes that cause problems in the feminine hygiene sprays.

Deodorant Pads and Tampons

At no time does a woman worry more about feminine odors than during a menstrual period. Appealing to that concern, pad and tampon manufacturers came up with what seemed like a dandy idea—add a deodorant or masking perfume to their products.

The only problem is, these additives can cause all the same problems that vaginal sprays and towelettes do, from skin irritations to allergic reactions. Deodorant tampons are particularly worthless because menstrual blood has no odor until it's exposed to air. You don't need extra chemicals and perfumes inside you.

The solution to menstrual odors? We hate to sound like a broken record, but regular washing plus frequent changes of sanitary products is the simplest and safest way.

Trich or Treat?

Here comes one of those choices where it seems you just can't win. Should you put up with a form of vaginitis known as trichomoniasis that causes vaginal itching and a green or grayish discharge with a foul smell and that may lead to urinary tract problems. . . .

. . . or do you get rid of it with the only medicine available for the problem, a very effective drug called metronidazole (Flagyl), which—says Ralph Nader's Health Research Group—may cause cancer, genetic mutations and birth defects?

You won't have to make the choice if you can obtain relief from twice-a-day baths, douches every other week using a tablespoon of white vinegar in a quart of warm water and avoiding tight undergarments.

However, if this method doesn't do the trick, there is a safe way to use Flagyl, according to Yehudi Felman, M.D., director of New York City's bureau of VD control. The key is the amount of time you take it. Dr. Felman says that no long-term side effects should be caused by a *1-week* course of treatment (for *both* partners). He also urges anyone taking the drug to completely avoid alcohol, which can interact with Flagyl to produce unpleasant side effects.

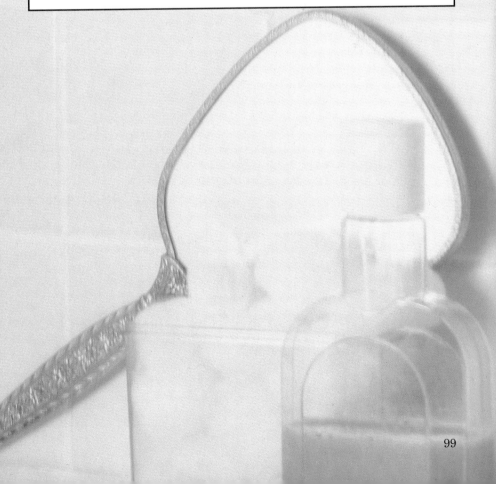

Since weekly treatment with the tincture is necessary to completely kill all the viruses causing the warts, you might consider having them removed another way. Freezing with liquid nitrogen is a sensible alternative to and much more popular than the old method of burning them off. But whatever method your doctor chooses, be patient, since Dr. Felman warns that everyone's recovery time is different. Some people will stop getting new warts after 4 visits; some others may need 40.

DIET AND WEIGHT LOSS

"Lose Weight Fast." So say the advertising claims that echo every pudgy person's dreams. In the quest for a slender body some ten million people swallow this hope each day in the form of capsules, pills, candy, gums or drops.

Although the effectiveness of these pills has been questioned in some quarters, the biggest concerns raised by consumer groups and researchers alike are the side effects. And high blood pressure, central nervous system disorders and even psychotic disorders head the list.

The villain in all the controversy over the diet pills is the active ingredient phenylpropanolamine (PPA). PPA affects the hypothalamus, a portion of the brain that regulates the appetite. Apparently PPA has the strength to persuade your appetite that you're not hungry. So fooled, you eat less and lose weight.

In one study, PPA diet pills were compared with placebos (harmless blank pills) in two groups of obese patients. After four weeks, the median weight loss was 5½ pounds for the PPA patients and 4 pounds for the placebo group.

Another active ingredient—benzocaine—which is found in chewing gum and candy-type diet aids, also has been found to be helpful in suppressing the appetite.

A New Drug Treatment for Anorexics

Therapy that acts directly on the brain is producing amazing results in those suffering from the self-starvation disorder known as anorexia nervosa.

"Our success rate so far in those who can be truly classified as anorexic has been 100 percent," says James Parsons, M.D., a psychiatrist who practices the therapy at his one-of-a-kind eating disorders clinic in Melbourne, Florida.

The rationale behind the treatment is simple. "It's been known since 1977 that anorexics have high levels of cortisol, an adrenal hormone in the brain," explains Dr. Parsons.

"When a woman deprives herself of nutrients over a period of time, her body eventually opens the cortisol spigot, providing her with an artificial infusion of energy. The release of cortisol results in brain swelling, which impairs frontal lobe function. The prevailing chemical reaction causes afflicted persons to actually have a distorted image of themselves and to believe they are extremely overweight, when in fact they are becoming severely emaciated," says Dr. Parsons.

Dr. Parsons and his colleagues decided to see what would happen when they combined low doses of already existing drugs and vitamins. Prescribed for a variety of unrelated ailments, they have one thing in common: They lower cortisol levels.

Dr. Parsons says his treatment combines such things as ulcer medication, local anesthetics and certain antihistamines, plus vitamin C and tryptophan. "They all are given in very low doses so they won't be toxic," he says.

The result? "It works like charm," he claims.

Benzocaine is a topical anesthetic usually found in throat lozenges. In theory, the benzocaine numbs the taste buds to keep you from enjoying the taste of food. People who can't taste their food are unlikely to heap their plates or take second helpings.

A QUESTION OF SAFETY

Just because these diet aids are sold over the counter doesn't mean they are completely safe. Although nothing more harmful than a rash has been attributed to benzocaine, there have been reports of serious side effects from PPA, even when taken as directed.

Most notable is a study conducted on 72 healthy medical students at the University of Melbourne in Australia. The students were divided into two groups. One group took diet pills containing 85 milligrams of PPA per capsule while the other group was given a placebo. Blood pressure reached a peak 1½ to 3 hours after the diet pills were given. In 12 out of 37 who took the drug, diastolic pressure rose to dangerously high levels. Three people actually required treatment. Because of the alarming blood pressure effects, researchers decided to substitute a diet pill containing only 50 milligrams of PPA. But it, too, was found to induce high blood pressure.

It was this study that convinced the U.S. Food and Drug Administration to reconsider the dosage of 150 milligrams sanctioned by its investigative committee. Right now the FDA says that 75 milligrams of PPA is the maximum dose allowed in 24 hours for any diet pill.

Side effects, unfortunately, are not limited to soaring blood pressure. They also include problems with mind and mood. "The wide use of phenylpropanolamine as a decongestant for colds, hay fever and sinusitis, plus its increasing use as an oral over-the-counter anorexic agent, indicates a need to increase our awareness of its possible serious psychiatric side effects," says Charles B. Schaffer, M.D., of the University of California School of Medicine.

In one recent study, seven women experienced symptoms ranging from tremor and restlessness to agitation

<table>
<tr><td>

Snooze 'N' Lose?
Easy Weight-Loss Scheme Only a Dream

"If people want to take cough syrup for their bunions, there's not much we can do to stop them." That pretty much sums up how one FDA official feels about the usefulness of the new wave in easy weight-loss schemes—the amino acids L-ornithine and L-arginine. And he by no means stands alone in his opinion.

The theory behind the claim—made popular by California health consultant Durk Pearson and Sandy Shaw in their book *Life Extension*—is that ornithine and arginine, when taken on an empty stomach and before bedtime, trigger the release of growth hormones that will help you burn fat *and* build muscle—all while you sleep.

But most doctors don't agree with this claim. In fact, even if the pills *do* work as claimed, there is some concern about their safety.

"If arginine and ornithine work—if they do raise growth hormone levels—then people shouldn't use them," says nutrition expert Alan Gaby, M.D., of Baltimore, Maryland. "Elevation of growth hormone levels can cause diabetes. The bottom line," says Dr. Gaby, "is that there is no solid research on the effects of arginine and ornithine, and I would like to see more studies on their safety before I would tell anyone to take them."

</td></tr>
</table>

and hallucinations after taking just one PPA diet tablet. One medical journal reported on a 13-year-old girl who suffered high blood pressure and a generalized seizure after taking a capsule containing 75 milligrams of PPA plus 200 milligrams of caffeine (a common ingredient in some OTC diet pills). In Sweden, 61 cases of central nervous system disturbance were reported after taking PPA. And in the United States, episodes of paranoia, homicidal behavior, psychosis, mania, hallucination and attempted suicide have also been reported—all after taking diet pills containing PPA.

"The risk of these anorexic agents as diet aids may outweigh their benefits," warns Dr. Schaffer, "because there is no reliable evidence that PPA can help obese patients achieve long-term weight reduction."

Our advice: Stay away from PPA.

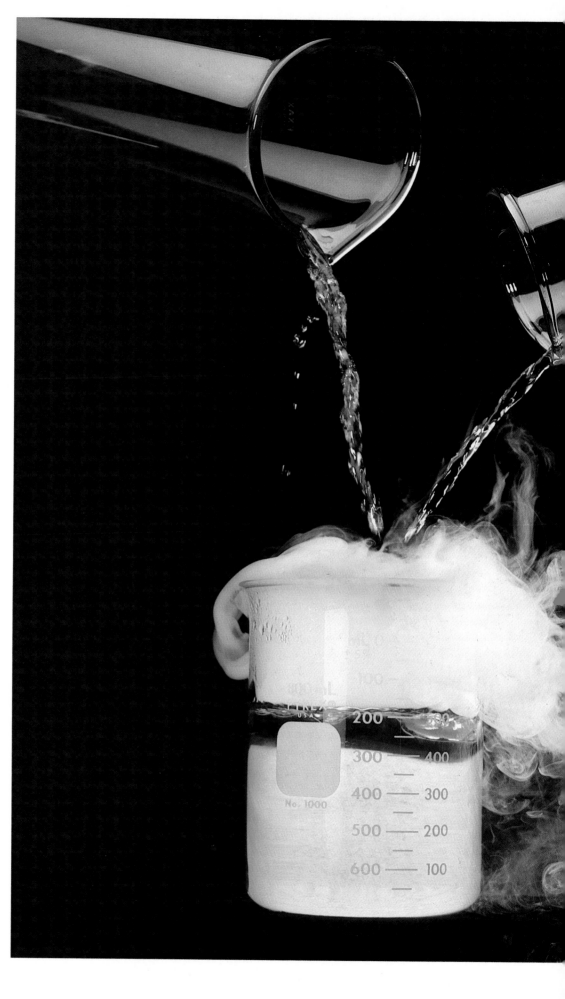

7

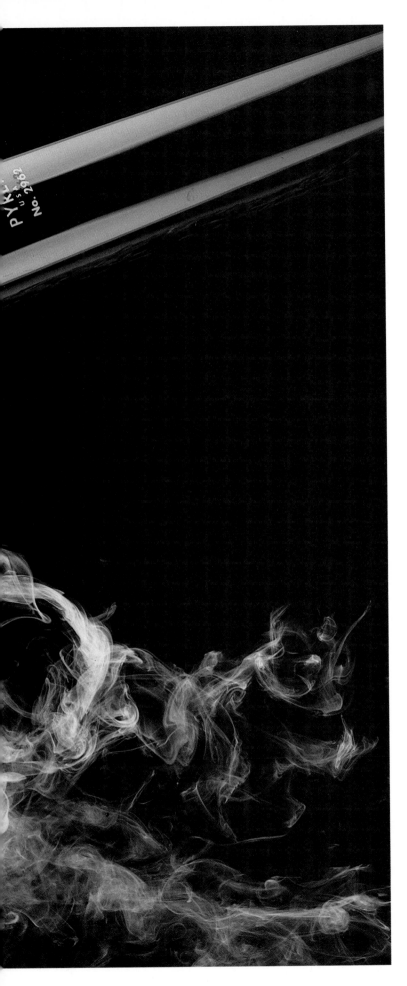

Preventing Side Effects

A complete guide to the side effects of the 51 most prescribed drugs: how to spot them and—if possible—stop them.

He was a successful 32-year-old lawyer revving up for a brilliant career in politics. But suddenly his future didn't look so bright—his doctor diagnosed dangerously high blood pressure and put him on medication to control it. He hadn't felt too bad before, but then he started taking the pills. He became sluggish, drowsy, depressed—not exactly winning attributes for an ambitious young man.

She was an active older woman who loved the outdoors and frequently roamed meadows and woods. Unfortunately, she roamed too close to a beehive and was stung several times. Her doctor of 20 years gave her a prescription for a new antiallergy medication and she went to bed pain free. In the middle of the night, she woke up to a room spinning like a top, feeling sick to her stomach.

Both of these people were victims of one of the most common medical ailments of all: side effects. These include *any* unwanted effects produced by a drug. They occur hundreds of times a day, millions of times a year, and are usually brought on simply by taking prescribed or over-the-counter medication. They also can result from taking too much or too little of a drug, or from mixing it with other drugs or even certain foods, drinks or nutritional supplements.

COULD IT HAPPEN TO YOU?

Any drug can have a side effect, even a safe, widely used workhorse like aspirin. Luckily, few have the chamber-of-horrors severity of drugs like DES or thalidomide. Common side effects can include upset stomach, nausea, vomiting, diar-

Injections: Not Just a Pain in the Rump

Ouch! Those shots in tender spots really hurt. Now there's evidence they do more than make you sore: They can actually cause tissue decay and paralysis.

German doctors studying a number of suspected malpractice cases found that 90 involved intramuscular (buttock) injections. Among these, most had severe and permanent disability. In 26 cases, flesh decayed in the area injected, causing acute pain. In 23 cases, the injections led to paralysis of the sciatic nerve, which runs down the leg. Eighty-two percent of these cases were due to injection of drugs to reduce fever or inflammatory diseases such as arthritis. The study concluded that oral doses are just as effective.

rhea and other gastrointestinal problems; fatigue, lethargy or similar responses of the central nervous system; or skin rashes, as well as other allergic reactions.

Could a side effect happen to you? Consider these statistics: 75 million of us take one or more drugs every week and spend over $11 billion annually for them. According to Lowell Levin, Ed.D., professor of public health at Yale University School of Medicine, at least 5 million Americans might have an adverse drug reaction within any given year.

A recent report from the annual Symposium on Drug Allergy says that 1 of every 30 hospitalizations in the United States is the result of a drug reaction.

These frightening statistics suggest that problems stemming from the use of various medications are reaching epidemic levels. Like every health problem, this epidemic has a name: iatrogenic disease, illness accidentally created by medical treatment.

How can a drug that actually makes you feel worse be handed out by physicians who are trying to make you feel better? The answer is complicated—complicated by unforeseen individual reactions, complicated by side effects that don't show up until years after a drug has been on the market, and complicated even more by the traditional relationship between doctor and patient. The road to a side effect starts in a drug company's high-tech lab and ends in your doctor's examining room.

PAVED WITH GOOD INTENTIONS

Drug testing begins with the manufacturers who study new drugs for safety and effectiveness. However, these drugs are infrequently tested on the elderly—by far the largest group of drug users. Moreover, those who take the experimental drug are not monitored over long periods. If, at the end of the trial period, the drug seems safe, it is submitted to the U.S. Food and Drug Administration for approval. Once this government agency determines that the

drug's benefits outweigh its risks, it okays the drug and a physician is free to prescribe it. While a doctor might know of a drug's side effects, he may not warn you of these potential dangers. As a result, you and your doctor become unknowing participants in a continuing study of the drug's effects.

Joe Graedon, a pharmacologist who's written three books on drugs and side effects, says, "I think a physician sincerely wants to do well by his patient. He doesn't want to imply that what can help can hurt you, and he might be afraid that if he tells a patient of a drug's side effects, the patient won't take it. Also, many physicians are afraid that if they mention side effects, the patient will experience them psychosomatically; if he mentions headache or nausea, the patient will *get* headache or nausea."

What can you do to break down this wall of well-intentioned silence? Ask questions. Be diplomatic, but get answers. One survey showed a shockingly low 2 to 4 percent of patients ever muster up the courage to ask their doctors about side effects.

TAKING CHARGE OF TAKING DRUGS

Since you are the person taking the medication, you must assume the responsibility to find out about it. Here are some questions you might ask.

What Will This Drug Do for My Condition? What kind of medicine is it? How is it supposed to help? Will it actually cure the problem or only provide temporary relief?

Richard G. Fried, M.D., a Pennsylvania family physician, says, "A patient should ask his doctor, 'Is this medication symptomatic or curative? Is it going to relieve symptoms that might go away anyway, or actually help to heal my condition?'"

Is the Dose Tailored to My Body's Needs? Each individual has a different metabolism, and everyone's system slows with age. Did your physician consider your individuality and possible allergic reactions? Is the dosage at the lowest level possible to achieve a therapeutic effect? Will the dosage have to be changed in the future?

What Are the Side Effects and Interactions? Does the drug have any effects I should watch out for? Is it all right to drive or do other demanding tasks when I'm taking it? Is it all right to take with other medicines I might need? Are there any unusual reactions with food or beverages, especially alcohol?

Says Dr. Levin, "We must be prepared for some degree of risk in drug taking, but if we're better informed and know what the risk is, the appearance of the side effect won't be so unexpected and provoke so much anxiety."

How Should I Take It? Does this drug work best on a full or an empty stomach? Should I take it with milk, water or some other liquid? How often should I take it? At what time of day? What should I do if I miss a dose? What should I do if I accidentally take an overdose?

Lawrence H. Block, Ph.D., professor of pharmaceutics at the Duquesne University School of Pharmacy, Pittsburgh, says, "The doctor must make certain the instructions for using a drug are *absolutely* clear, and reinforce those directions not only verbally but in writing."

How Long Should I Take It? How long do I need to take this medication? Will I need to taper the dose when I stop? What should I do if I run out? When do I need to see the doctor again, and what will he want to know then?

Will This Drug Affect My Nutrition? Even if you eat a wholesome diet, the drug you're taking may keep you from getting enough of certain nutrients. William H. Lee, Ph.D., a New York City nutritionist, says many drugs interfere with basic nutrition in a "domino effect."

"The loss of one nutrient could mean the loss of others down the line," he says. "For instance, if a drug interferes with folate, it also will interfere with vitamin B_{12}, and

eventually your RNA. By increasing your intake of folate, some more might get through. If you don't increase it, you're guaranteeing it won't get through."

Dr. Lee recommends that you always ask your physician if a drug will affect your nutrition and how it will do so. If he doesn't know, ask him to find out, or look it up in nutrition books yourself. (But don't take large amounts of any nutrient to make up for these losses without your doctor's approval.)

In summary, Dr. Fried says he doesn't believe in telling the patient about every possible side effect. "I don't go through a whole litany of every reported side effect. I *do* tell the patient a few of the most common and most serious side effects they're likely to encounter, then make it clear to that patient he can call me at the first sign of a side effect."

After learning about what to expect from your medication, you also have to watch for other side effects no one told you about. For example, a drug can be less effective if you smoke or take laxatives or antacids. In that case, your doctor might have to increase the dosage.

Even after all these painstaking efforts, you still may experience an *allergic* reaction to a drug. Possible symptoms include rash, nausea, vomiting, diarrhea, extreme sensitivity to light, burning, itching, dizziness and fatigue. If your reaction is severe, get help immediately. In extreme cases, your body could go into anaphylactic shock, which can be fatal.

Does learning about a drug's possible side efects have to be a lot of trouble? Not at all. The chart that follows tells you the main side effects of the 51 most frequently prescribed drugs, as well as how they interact with food, beverages and other medications. A second chart lists the sexual side effects of many commonly prescribed drugs. Take time to review the charts for information about the drugs you and members of your family are taking. Also use them as a basis for questions to ask your doctor. A keen curiosity on your part is the first step in a "healthy" skepticism that will help you use medicines wisely.

Drug Side Effects

	Drug	Use	Possible Side Effects	
A	**Achromycin V, other tetracyclines**	Treatment of infection	May cause discolored tongue, sore mouth and throat, nausea, vomiting, diarrhea; may stain developing teeth; may result in superinfections. Tetracyclines may kill off beneficial as well as harmful bacteria and cause fungus infections. Dramatic weight loss, anemia, liver failure have occurred.	
	Aldomet	Control of high blood pressure; reduction of fluid retention	May cause drowsiness, lethargy, headache, dizziness, weakness, light-headedness, stuffy nose, dry mouth the first few weeks of therapy. Bloating and weight gain are possible. After prolonged use, episodes may occur when the drug's effect is abruptly lost; these may be accompanied by tremors and stiffness.	
	Aldoril	Control of high blood pressure; reduction of fluid retention	*See* Aldomet	
	Amoxil	Treatment of infection	May cause discolored tongue, nausea, vomiting, diarrhea, anemia; may result in superinfections.	
	Antivert	Relief of nausea, vomiting and dizziness of motion sickness	May cause drowsiness, dryness of mouth, nose and throat. Use caution when driving or operating machinery. Overdose may cause stupor, confusion, loss of coordination and muscle tremors, leading to coma and possible death.	
	Ativan	Relief of anxiety	May cause clumsiness, drowsiness, dizziness, lethargy, lack of coordination, memory loss, confusion. May cause increased sedation and hangover effect if used continuously. May affect all levels of mental and physical performance; use caution when driving or operating machinery. Prolonged use may result in liver damage, a reduction of white blood cells (thus reducing ability to fight off infections) and addiction. Overdose may cause marked drowsiness, weakness, feeling of drunkenness, staggering; large overdose may cause tremors and lead to deep sleep or coma.	
B	**Bactrim, Bactrim DS**	Treatment of infection	May cause headache, fatigue, dizziness, weakness, loss of appetite, nausea, vomiting, diarrhea, superinfections, itchy rash; may darken urine. Prolonged use in large amounts may result in enlarged thyroid gland.	
	Benadryl capsules and tablets	Relief of symptoms of hay fever, allergies, motion sickness, Parkinson's disease	May cause sedation, drowsiness, dizziness, impaired coordination, dryness of nose, mouth and throat, nausea, constipation. Prolonged use may result in bone marrow damage, nerve damage and the destruction of red blood cells, leading to anemia.	
C	**Ceclor**	Treatment of infection	Usually, none. Diarrhea, nausea and vomiting have been noted in about 2 percent of patients. Prolonged use may result in superinfections.	

Possible Interactions			
Food/Drink	**Nutrients**	**Alcohol/Smoking**	**Other Medications**
For best results, take 1 hour before or 2 hours after eating. Avoid dairy products, especially milk, for 1 hour before and 2 hours after each dose.	Interferes with absorption of calcium, iron, magnesium and zinc. Those on vitamin A therapy should be aware that this drug increases vitamin A absorption.	Avoid alcohol; may cause liver damage.	Decreases the effects of penicillin; may decrease the effectiveness of oral contraceptives. Antacids and iron/mineral supplements decrease tetracycline's effectiveness.
Works best when taken with meals. Drink enough water to satisfy thirst. Avoid natural licorice, which can lower the concentration of potassium in the bloodstream and cause dangerous heart rhythms.	Interferes with absorption of folate, iron and vitamin B_{12}.	Avoid alcohol; exaggerates Aldomet's effects, further lowering blood pressure.	Diuretics and other high blood pressure medications increase effects. Amphetamines and diet pills decrease effects. MAO inhibitors may dangerously elevate blood pressure.
Take with food 6 hours before bedtime. Avoid natural licorice. Reduce sodium, increase potassium in diet.	*See* Aldomet	*See* Aldomet	*See* Aldomet
Take 1 hour before or 2 hours after eating.	None	Alcohol may irritate the stomach.	Erythromycin, tetracycline and antacids decrease effectiveness.
Take with food or liquid to lessen stomach irritation.	None	Avoid alcohol; may cause rapid sedation, coma and death.	Taken with sedatives, tranquilizers, antidepressants, narcotics and other drugs that depress the central nervous system, the effects of both are increased, with potentially fatal effects.
Caffeine may decrease calming action.	None	Avoid alcohol completely; may cause heavy sedation. Smoking reduces Ativan's effects, proportional to the amount smoked.	Tagamet may delay elimination of Ativan from the body, causing excess sedation. Ativan increases the effects of high blood pressure medication and may cause a dangerous lowering of blood pressure. Increases the effects of drugs that depress the central nervous system like antihistamines, narcotics, sleeping pills and antidepressants, and may lead to deep sedation, seizures, coma and possible death. With anticonvulsants, Ativan may change seizure frequency and severity.
Take after eating and drink at least 2 quarts of water a day to prevent or lessen stomach irritation.	Interferes with absorption of vitamins C and K and folate. May cause kidney damage if taken with vitamin C supplements.	Increases the effects of alcohol.	Dangerous when taken with anticonvulsants. Aspirin and arthritis drugs may increase effects. Risk of abnormal bleeding and bruising increased if taken with diuretics. Low blood sugar may occur with antidiabetics. Bactrim decreases the effects of penicillin and other antibiotics.
Take after eating to lessen stomach irritation.	None	Avoid alcohol completely; causes greatly increased sedation.	Increases the effects of many drugs that depress the central nervous system such as narcotics, antidepressants, barbituates, sedatives and tranquilizers, causing over-sedation. Benadryl may decrease the effects of cortisone drugs.
Take 1 hour before or 2 hours after eating.	Decreases absorption of vitamin K.	Avoid alcohol.	Taken with anticoagulants, increases blood-thinning effects.

(continued)

	Drug	Use	Possible Side Effects	
C	**Clinoril**	Relief of arthritis pain	May cause dizziness, pain, indigestion, nausea, vomiting, diarrhea, constipation, headaches. Prolonged use may result in eye damage, reduced hearing, sore throat, fever, weight gain, mild anemia.	
	Corgard	Control of high blood pressure, angina	Those with hay fever or asthma should not take Corgard. Lethargy, fatigue, dry mouth and skin, tingling, cold and numbness in hands and feet may result from drop in blood pressure; diarrhea, nausea are common. Prolonged use may reduce heart muscle strength, weaken heart contractions and increase risk of heart failure.	
D	**Darvocet-N 100**	Relief of pain	May cause drowsiness, light-headedness, constipation, difficult urination. Overdose may decrease heart rate and respiration, leading to coma, convulsions and death. Prolonged use may result in addiction and anemia.	
	Diabinese	Control of diabetes	May cause abnormally low blood sugar, dizziness, diarrhea, loss of appetite, nausea, indigestion.	
	Dilantin	Prevention of seizures	May cause dizziness, drowsiness, rapid and uncontrollable jerking of the eyes, discoloration of urine, vomiting, constipation, nausea, lessening of sense of taste. Large overdose may cause deep sleep, lowering of blood pressure, slow, shallow breathing and eventual coma. Prolonged use may result in lymph gland enlargement, weakened bones, liver damage, bleeding and swelling of gums and nerve tissue damage that may progress to loss of coordination and strength.	
	Dimetapp	Relief of allergy symptoms	May cause drowsiness, dizziness, nausea, dryness of mouth, nose and throat. Moderate overdose may cause excitement, loss of coordination, hallucinations; large overdose may cause tremors, spasms, weak and rapid pulse, shallow breathing, stupor and eventual coma. Prolonged use may result in bone marrow damage, nerve damage and tardive dyskinesia. Dimetapp may cause or aggravate high blood pressure. Loses effectiveness if used regularly.	
	Donnatal	Relief of irritable bowel pain	May cause dizziness, drowsiness, rapid heartbeat, confusion, delirium, mental sluggishness, dryness of mouth, nose and throat, constipation, nausea, vomiting. Overdose may cause stupor, coma and death. Prolonged use may result in addiction, as well as chronic constipation, fecal impaction, anemia and a lowering of body temperature, making exposure to cold dangerous.	

Possible Interactions			
Food/Drink	**Nutrients**	**Alcohol/Smoking**	**Other Medications**
Most effective when taken 1 hour before or 2 hours after eating.	None	Alcohol increases irritating effects on the stomach, increasing risk of stomach bleeding and ulcers.	Aspirin, barbiturates and arthritis drugs decrease effectiveness and increase risk of stomach ulcer. Clinoril may increase the effects of some antibiotics, requiring a reduction of their dosage.
Take with meals or immediately afterward. Avoid natural licorice. Reduce sodium intake.	None	Alcohol may exaggerate Corgard's ability to lower blood pressure and may increase sedation.	Taken with quinidine, may cause excessive slowing of the heart. With digitalis, may affect heart rate and reduce digitalis's effects. Dangerously low blood pressure could result if taken with other high blood pressure medications. Corgard increases the effect of antidiabetics, causing or prolonging low blood sugar. Corgard exaggerates reserpine's effects, causing sedation, depression and low blood pressure. Drugs that depress the central nervous system may cause dangerous sedation. Corgard decreases the effects of antihistamines and anti-inflammatory drugs like Benadryl, aspirin and cortisone.
Take with liquid.	None	Avoid alcohol completely; causes increased sedation. Smoking reduces effectiveness.	All central nervous system depressants like sedatives, tranquilizers and anti-depressants increase sedative effects. May interfere with tetracycline's effects. Taken with acetaminophen over a long time, Darvocet may cause liver damage.
Take with liquid or food to lessen stomach irritation. Abnormally low blood sugar, coma and possible death may result from inadequate diet.	None	Avoid alcohol; may cause severe headache, abdominal cramps, nausea, vomiting and possible death.	May increase the effects of sedatives and sulfa drugs. Effects are decreased by major tranquilizers, cortisone drugs, estrogen, oral contraceptives, diuretics and thyroid drugs. Risk of drastic lowering of blood sugar if taken with aspirin, MAO inhibitors and certain high blood pressure drugs, antibiotics and pain relievers. Beta blockers (Inderal and Corgard) increase risk of high *and* low blood sugar. Steroid and anticonvulsant drugs may increase blood sugar.
Take with food or milk to reduce risk of nausea.	Interferes with absorption of vitamin D and folate. May need added folate to prevent anemia.	Alcohol may reduce effectiveness.	Sulfa drugs, aspirin in large doses, major and minor tranquilizers, estrogen and Ritalin all increase effects. Dilantin increases the effects of beta blockers, diuretics, high blood pressure drugs, digitalis, thyroid drugs and sedatives. Dilantin decreases the effects of oral contraceptives and cortisone drugs.
Take with food, milk or water.	None	Avoid alcohol; may cause excessive sedation.	Central nervous system depressants like antidepressants, sedatives and tranquilizers may cause excessive sedation. Beta blockers increase Dimetapp's effects. Dimetapp decreases the effects of cortisone drugs and oral anticoagulants.
Take with liquid or food to lessen stomach irritation.	Avoid large doses of vitamin C; decreases effectiveness.	Avoid alcohol.	Antidepressants, antihistamines and other central nervous system depressants greatly increase sedation. Taken with cortisone drugs and some major tranquilizers, may cause elevation in internal eye pressure. Donnatal decreases effects of cortisone drugs, digitalis, tetracycline, aspirin, beta blockers and oral contraceptives.

(continued)

	Drug	Use	Possible Side Effects	
D	**Dyazide**	Control of high blood pressure; treatment of bloating associated with congestive heart failure as well as cirrhosis of the liver and kidney disease	May cause dryness of mouth, nausea, vomiting. Prolonged use may cause retention of potassium, resulting in alteration of heart rhythm and performance.	
E	**E.E.S.**	Treatment of infection	High-dose therapy may cause superinfections.	
	Elavil	Relief of depression	May cause headache, insomnia, dryness of mouth and unpleasant taste, constipation, diarrhea, nausea, indigestion, craving for sweets, fatigue, weakness. Avoid all hazardous or demanding jobs. Overdose may cause extreme drowsiness, hallucinations, drop in body temperature, tremors; large overdose may cause convulsions, then coma, then death. Mild withdrawal symptoms may occur after prolonged use.	
	Empirin with codeine	Relief of pain	May cause dizziness, flushed face, difficult urination, tiredness. Prolonged use may cause ringing in ears, nausea, stomach pain, heartburn, ulcers, liver and kidney damage, vomiting, weakness, constipation. Overdose can slow breathing, leading to coma and death. May be habit forming.	
F	**Feldene**	Relief of arthritis symptoms	May cause indigestion, nausea, water retention, dizziness, headache, rash.	
	Fiorinal	Relief of headache pain	May cause drowsiness, dizziness, lethargy, hangover, light-headedness, nausea, vomiting, flatulence, sweating, flushing. Prolonged use may cause anemia, drop in body temperature, depression, kidney damage and possible dependency. Large overdose may cause coma and death.	
H	**HydroDIURIL**	Control of high blood pressure; reduction of water retention	May cause loss of appetite, gastrointestinal irritation, nausea, vomiting, light-headedness upon arising, increased blood levels of sugar and uric acid. Prolonged use may result in impaired balance of water, salt and potassium, diabetes in predisposed people, lifelong physical dependency on high blood pressure drugs.	
I	**Inderal**	Control of high blood pressure, angina, other heart problems	May cause dizziness, drowsiness, lethargy, fatigue, cold or tingling hands and feet, numbness, dryness of mouth and skin. Overdose may cause slow pulse, weakness, drop in blood pressure, convulsions, coma. Prolonged use reduces the reserve of heart muscle strength.	

Possible Interactions			
Food/Drink	**Nutrients**	**Alcohol/Smoking**	**Other Medications**
Avoid natural licorice, which may cause cramps, numbness, nausea, vomiting.	Interferes with absorption of potassium, zinc, folate, calcium and sodium.	Avoid alcohol; dramatically lowers blood pressure.	Increases effects of other high blood pressure drugs but decreases those of antidiabetics and gout drugs. Antidepressants can lower blood pressure excessively and may be fatal. Digitalis and cortisone drugs may cause dangerous heart irregularities.
Food interferes with absorption. Take 1 hour before or 2 hours after eating. Do not take with milk.	None	Avoid alcohol; may increase chance of liver damage.	Increases effects of asthma medications. Decreases penicillin's effects.
Take with food or liquid.	None	Avoid alcohol; results in excessive intoxication. Smoking may decrease effectiveness.	Taken with thyroids and quinidine, heart rhythms are impaired. Dangerous sedation may occur with drugs that depress the central nervous system. Barbiturates may decrease effectiveness. Elavil decreases the effects of high blood pressure drugs and may cause delirium with Placidyl. With MAO inhibitors, may cause fever, delirium, convulsions and acute psychosis. Certain diuretics increase Elavil's effects.
Take with liquid.	None	Avoid alcohol; increases central nervous system depression and causes excessive intoxication.	Taken with any central nervous system depressant, may cause increased sedation and possible coma. Decreases effects of gout drugs and lowers blood sugar with antidiabetics. Increases effects of cortisone drugs and increases risk of ulcers and stomach bleeding. With penicillin, effects of both drugs are increased. Barbiturates decrease effects. Empirin with codeine increases the effects of anticonvulsants. Codeine prolongs stomach emptying, thus hindering absorption and effectiveness of any oral drug.
None	None	None	Taken with aspirin, Feldene's effectiveness is decreased by as much as 20 percent.
Take with liquid or food to lessen stomach irritation.	None	Avoid alcohol; may cause oversedation, stupor and coma.	Sedatives, narcotics, tranquilizers and other drugs that depress the central nervous system increase sedation. Cortisone and arthritis drugs increase risk of ulcers, Fiorinal decreases effects of some antibiotics and anti-inflammatories, cortisone drugs, digitalis and tricyclic antidepressants.
Take with meals 6 or more hours before bedtime. Avoid natural licorice. Increase intake of foods high in potassium.	Raises calcium levels in blood, lowers levels of sodium, potassium, phosphorus and magnesium	*See* Dyazide	*See* Dyazide
Take with meals or after eating. Avoid natural licorice. Reduce sodium intake and calorie consumption.	None	Avoid alcohol; may further depress blood pressure and cause increased sedation. Smoking reduces effectiveness, may cause irregular heartbeat.	Taken with quinidine or digitalis, may slow heartbeat. Inderal increases effects of other high blood pressure medications. May increase effects of antidiabetics, with lowering of blood sugar. Inderal may block the effects of aspirin and cortisone drugs, and can cause dangerous oversedation with central nervous system depressants. Inderal decreases effects of allergy medications. Anticonvulsants taken with Inderal increase the effects of both drugs.

(continued)

	Drug	Use	Possible Side Effects	
I	**Indocin**	Relief of symptoms of arthritis, other inflammatory diseases	May cause dizziness, headache, ringing in ears, nausea, indigestion, heartburn. May hide symptoms of infection. Prolonged use may result in eye damage, hearing loss, sore throat, fever, weight gain. Overdose may cause stomach irritation, nausea, vomiting, diarrhea, confusion, agitation; large overdose may cause coma or hemorrhage of the stomach or intestines.	
	Isordil	Control of angina	May cause nausea, vomiting, rapid heartbeat, headaches that can be severe and persistent, flushed face and neck, light-headedness upon arising. Overdose may cause fainting and shortness of breath; large overdose may cause coma. Prolonged use may cause the drug to lose effectiveness.	
K	**Keflex**	Treatment of infection	May cause rash, redness, itching. Prolonged use may result in superinfections.	
L	**Lanoxin**	Control of high blood pressure	May cause loss of appetite, diarrhea, nausea, vomiting, irregular heartbeat. Moderate overdose may cause loss of appetite, excess salivation, nausea, vomiting, diarrhea; large overdose may cause serious heart irregularities, internal bleeding, drowsiness, headaches, hallucinations, convulsions. Lanoxin has a narrow margin of safety; carry medical alert I.D.	
	Lasix Oral	Control of high blood pressure; reduction of water retention	May cause dizziness, light-headedness and increased levels of blood sugar and uric acid, affecting diabetes and gout. Prolonged use may impair balance of water, salt and potassium in body and may cause diabetes in predisposed people. Overdose may cause weakness, fatigue, drowsiness, leading to deep sleep, weak and rapid pulse, cardiac arrest.	
	Lopressor	Control of high blood pressure	May cause depression, shortness of breath, diarrhea. *Also see* Inderal	
M	**Minipress**	Control of high blood pressure	May cause drowsiness, dizziness, light-headedness upon arising, heart palpitations, headache, weakness, nausea.	
	Motrin	Relief of pain	May cause dizziness, headache, nausea, stomach pain, heartburn, rash. Prolonged use may result in eye damage, hearing loss, sore throat, fever, weight gain.	
N	**Naldecon**	Relief of allergy symptoms, congestion	May cause drowsiness, nervousness, headache, dizziness, pallor, insomnia, rapid heartbeat, rise in blood pressure for predisposed people. Overdose may cause muscle tremors, spasms, severe anxiety, delirium. Prolonged use may result in more severe congestion after treatment.	

Possible Interactions			
Food/Drink	**Nutrients**	**Alcohol/Smoking**	**Other Medications**
Take with meals or after eating to lessen stomach irritation.	May interfere with absorption of vitamin C and amino acids. Increases blood levels of potassium.	Alcohol may increase risk of stomach bleeding and ulcers.	Aspirin inhibits effectiveness of Indocin, and together they increase risk of ulcers. Indocin increases effects of cortisone drugs, with increased risk of ulcers, and decreases the effects of certain drugs used to reduce swelling.
For best results, take 1 or 2 hours after eating.	None	Alcohol may cause dramatic drop in blood pressure.	Taken with high blood pressure drugs and tricyclic antidepressants, may cause excessive drop in blood pressure.
Take 1 hour before or 2 hours after eating.	Interferes with potassium uptake.	Avoid alcohol.	May increase the effects of anticoagulants; dosage adjustment may be necessary.
Take with meals to reduce nausea. If meals are high in dietary fiber, take 30 minutes before or 2 hours after eating. Avoid caffeine, natural licorice and herb teas. Reduce sodium intake and maintain adequate magnesium in diet.	Interferes with potassium absorption. Avoid high amounts of vitamin D supplements.	Nicotine may make monitoring of Lanoxin's effectiveness difficult.	Other high blood pressure medications, thyroid drugs, cortisone drugs, drugs used to reduce swelling, quinidine may cause loss of appetite, nausea, vomiting, confusion, blurred vision, sensitivity to light, unusual fatigue or weakness, headache, irregular or changed heartbeat. Barbiturates, laxatives and antacids decrease Lanoxin's effects.
Take with food, always several hours before bedtime. May raise cholesterol level. Eat plenty of foods rich in potassium and magnesium.	Decreases absorption of calcium, magnesium, potassium, sodium and chloride.	Avoid alcohol; may cause drastic drop in blood pressure. Smoking may decrease Lasix's effects.	Reduces effects of antidiabetics. May cause aspirin toxicity. Cortisone causes an excessive loss of potassium. Taken with Lasix Oral, digitalis causes dangerous heart rhythms. Sedatives and some antidepressants can dramatically lower blood pressure. Indocin decreases ability to reduce bloating.
See Inderal	None	*See* Inderal	*See* Inderal
None	None	Use alcohol with extreme caution; may cause dramatic drop in blood pressure.	Taken with antidepressants and antipsychotics, Minipress may cause agitation. With MAO inhibitors, may cause a drop in blood pressure. Nitroglycerin prolongs Minipress's effectiveness. Taken with high blood pressure drugs, Minipress increases effects of both drugs.
Take with food to lessen stomach irritation.	None	Alcohol causes increased risk of stomach bleeding and ulcers.	Taken with cortisone, gout drugs and aspirin, may cause increased chance of ulcers. With anticoagulants there is increased risk of bleeding. With thyroid medications, may cause rapid heartbeat, rise in blood pressure.
Take with food or water. Caffeine taken with Naldecon may cause nervousness and insomnia.	None	Limit alcohol; causes increased sedation.	Taken with tricyclic antidepressants, may cause rapid heartbeat, rise in blood pressure. With barbiturates, sedative-hypnotics and tranquilizers, may cause increased sedation. MAO inhibitors increase Naldecon's effects and cause a dangerous rise in blood pressure. Naldecon may decrease the effects of high blood pressure drugs. With digitalis, may cause serious heart rhythm disturbances.

(continued)

	Drug	Use	Possible Side Effects	
N	**Naprosyn**	Relief of arthritis and menstrual pain	May cause dizziness, headache, nausea, abdominal pain, tendency to bruise and bleed easily. Prolonged use may result in kidney or eye damage, sore throat, fever, weight gain. May mask infections.	
O	**Omnipen**	Treatment of infection	May cause discolored tongue; may result in superinfections. Do not use if allergic to penicillin. Those with mononucleosis may develop severe rash.	
P	**Penn-Vee K**	Treatment of infection	May cause dark, discolored tongue, other irritations of the mouth and tongue, possible nausea, vomiting, diarrhea; may increase risk of superinfections.	
	Persantine	Control of angina	May cause light-headedness, flushing. Overdose may cause marked drop in blood pressure with weak, rapid pulse, nausea, vomiting, cramps, diarrhea.	
	Premarin	Treatment of menstrual and menopausal discomfort and irregularities, weakened bones, prostate and breast cancer	May cause fluid retention and bloating, weight gain, breakthrough bleeding and other menstrual problems, increased susceptibility to yeast infections, loss of appetite, stomach cramps, nausea, diarrhea. Prolonged use may result in fibroid growth in the uterus, blood clots in the lung, heart, eye or leg, stroke, heart attack. Premarin contains estrogen, which has been associated with a greater risk of cancer of the uterus, gallbladder disease and raised blood pressure.	
	Procardia	Control of angina	May cause fatigue, dizziness, nausea, weakness. Overdose may cause change in heart rate, unconsciousness, cardiac arrest.	
R	**Restoril**	Relief of insomnia	May cause clumsiness, drowsiness, dizziness, lethargy, confusion. Overdose may cause weakness, tremor, stupor, coma. Prolonged use may impair liver function and cause dependency.	
S	**Slow-K**	Replacement of potassium depleted by other drugs	May cause mild laxative effect.	
	Synthroid	Treatment of thyroid deficiencies	May cause tremors, headache, irritability, insomnia, appetite changes, weight loss, diarrhea, leg cramps, menstrual problems, fever, heat sensitivity, unusual sweating. Overdose may cause heart palpitations, irregular, rapid pulse.	

Possible Interactions			
Food/Drink	**Nutrients**	**Alcohol/Smoking**	**Other Medications**
Take with food to lessen stomach irritation.	None	Alcohol causes increased risk of stomach bleeding and ulcers.	Increases the effects of antibiotics, anticonvulsants and diabetes drugs. Aspirin decreases its effect, and aspirin and cortisone increase the risk of stomach ulcers. With thyroid medication, may cause rapid heartbeat, rise in blood pressure.
Take 1 hour before or 2 hours after eating.	None	Alcohol may cause stomach irritation.	Taken with erythromycin, tetracycline and sulfa drugs, may cause decreased effects of both drugs. May decrease effectiveness of oral contraceptives.
Take 1 hour before or 2 hours after eating. Blue cheese inhibits effects.	None	Alcohol occasionally may cause stomach irritation.	Aspirin, certain arthritis drugs and sulfa drugs increase penicillin's effects. Tetracycline, erythromycin and some other antibiotics decrease effects.
Take 1 hour before or 2 hours after eating.	None	Alcohol may cause dramatic drop in blood pressure.	Drastic lowering of blood pressure with high blood pressure medication. Aspirin increases Persantine's effect; dosage adjustment may be needed.
None	Depletes vitamin C, folate, calcium, magnesium and riboflavin. Increases levels of iron, vitamins A and E.	None	Taken with anticonvulsants, may cause greater risk of seizures. Unpredictable effect on antidiabetics, either increased or decreased blood sugar. Decreases effects of medications that lower cholesterol and thyroid drugs. Barbiturates decrease Premarin's effectiveness.
Most effective when taken 1 hour before or 2 hours after eating.	Large doses of vitamin D decrease effects.	Avoid alcohol; causes hazardous drop in blood pressure.	Procardia increases effects of anticonvulsant drugs and alters the effects of heart rhythm medication. High blood pressure drugs and diuretic drugs cause a dangerous decline in blood pressure. Procardia increases effects of digitalis. Sudden withdrawal from beta blockers may cause increased angina attacks.
None	None	Avoid alcohol; causes heavy sedation. Smoking increases Restoril's effects.	Taken with central nervous system depressants such as antihistamines, barbiturates, sleeping pills, antidepressants and narcotics, effects of both drugs are increased. With high blood pressure medication, may cause blood pressure to drop drastically. With MAO inhibitors, may cause convulsions, deep sedation and rage.
Take with food to lessen stomach irritation.	With prolonged use, slows absorption of vitamin B_{12} and may cause anemia.	Alcohol may cause stomach irritation.	Diuretics may cause a reduction in potassium. Some high blood pressure drugs may cause excessive potassium levels.
Take on an empty stomach to improve absorption. Members of the cabbage family (brussels sprouts, cabbage, cauliflower, kale, kohlrabi, rutabagas, turnips) and soybeans may interfere with long-term thyroid therapy.	None	None	Antidiabetics may need dosage adjustment. With tricyclic antidepressants, antidepressant effect is increased. Large, continuous doses of aspirin increase effects. Oral contraceptives decrease Synthroid's effects. Effects of digitalis are increased. Certain anticonvulsants increase Synthroid's effects. Cortisone drugs' effects may be decreased.

(continued)

T

Drug	Use	Possible Side Effects	
Tagamet	Treatment of stomach ulcers	May cause dizziness, muscular pain, mild diarrhea, rash. Prolonged use may result in liver damage, swelling and soreness of breast tissue in men.	
Tenormin	Control of high blood pressure	*See* Inderal	
Theo-Dur	Relief of asthma symptoms	May cause nervousness, nausea, vomiting, stomach pain, insomnia, headaches, irritability, stomach irritation.	
Timoptic	Treatment of glaucoma	May precipitate asthma and drop in blood pressure, with light-headedness, dizziness, drowsiness, numbness, tingling and cold hands and feet, dryness of mouth and skin. Overdose may cause severe respiratory and cardiac reactions, including death in asthmatics and those with heart problems.	
Tolinase	Control of diabetes	May cause dizziness, drowsiness, loss of appetite, diarrhea, nausea, stomach pain. If drug dosage is excessive or food intake too low, low blood sugar may result.	
Triavil	Relief of anxiety associated with depression	May cause restlessness, tremor, drowsiness, less perspiration, dryness of mouth and unpleasant taste, nasal congestion, muscle spasms of face and neck, unsteady gait, headache, insomnia, craving for sweets, fatigue, weakness, blurred and impaired vision, constipation, diarrhea, nausea, indigestion. Overdose may cause confusion, heart palpitations, stupor, convulsions, coma.	
Tylenol with codeine	Relief of pain	May cause dizziness, drowsiness, flushed face, unusual tiredness, light-headedness, nausea, vomiting, difficult urination, constipation.	

V

Valium	Relief of anxiety	*See* Ativan. Valium can accumulate in the body, causing increased sedation.	

Z

Zyloprim	Relief of gout; prevention of kidney stone formation.	May cause rash, hives, itching. Frequency and severity of gout attacks may increase during the first few weeks of treatment.	

	Possible Interactions		
Food/Drink	**Nutrients**	**Alcohol/Smoking**	**Other Medications**
For best results, take with food or milk. Caffeine drinks may increase acid secretion and reduce effectiveness.	None	Alcohol may increase stomach acidity and decrease effectiveness. Smoking decreases effectiveness.	May delay elimination of Valium from the body, causing increased sedation. Tagamet increases effects of digitoxin, penicillin, Theo-Dur, anticoagulants, quinidine and some asthma medications.
Take with food.	None	Avoid alcohol; may cause excessive blood pressure drop. Smoking may cause irregular heartbeat.	Taken with digitalis or quinidine, may cause slowing of heart rate. With other high blood pressure drugs, effects of both are increased. Decreases effectiveness of antihistamines, antidiabetics and anti-inflammatory drugs. May increase sedative effects of barbiturates, narcotics and reserpine.
Most effective when taken on an empty stomach, with 8 ounces of water. Where stomach irritation occurs, take with food. Avoid caffeine. Milk and dairy products and iron preparations should not be consumed within 2 hours of taking Theo-Dur.	Reduces absorption of calcium, iron, magnesium, zinc and amino acids. Reduces synthesis of potassium. Vitamin A supplements may present problems.	None	Increases effects of certain antibloating, high blood pressure drugs. Decreases effects of gout drugs. With reserpine, may cause rapid heartbeat. Erythromycin increases effects. With Inderal, effects of Theo-Dur are decreased.
None.	None	Alcohol causes excessive drop in blood pressure.	Anticonvulsants increase Timoptic's effects. With barbiturates, narcotics, and other central nervous system depressants, may cause increased sedation. Timoptic decreases the effectiveness of arthritis medications and antihistamines. With antidiabetics, beta blockers and high blood pressure drugs, Timoptic's effects are increased.
Tolinase is just one part of a total program for management of diabetes, not a substitute for a controlled diet.	None	Avoid alcohol; may cause severe headaches, nausea, vomiting, chest pain, shortness of breath, possible death. Smoking may reduce effectiveness.	Increases the effects of sleeping pills, antibiotics and tranquilizers. Aspirin, arthritis drugs, beta blockers, MAO inhibitors increase effects. Diuretics, thyroid drugs, major tranquilizers, estrogen, cortisone drugs, oral contraceptives and anticonvulsants all decrease effectiveness.
See Elavil	None	*See* Elavil	*See* Elavil
None	None	Avoid alcohol; codeine increases intoxicating effects.	Taken with other narcotics, as well as with sedatives, hypnotics, analgesics, tranquilizers or antidepressants, may cause increased sedation.
Take with food or water. Avoid caffeine.	*See* Ativan	*See* Ativan	*See* Ativan
Take after eating to lessen stomach irritation, nausea. Caffeine diminishes effectiveness. Increase fluid intake.	Taking iron supplements may lead to excessive iron levels in the body. Do not take with vitamin C supplements.	Avoid alcohol; may impair management of gout.	Taken with ampicillin, may cause skin rashes. Oral antidiabetics may increase uric acid elimination. Diuretics and high blood pressure drugs like Dyazide, Lasix Oral and Aldoril may decrease Zyloprim's effects.

Sexual Side Effects of Commonly Prescribed Drugs

Drug	Use	Increased (A) or Decreased (B) Sex Drive	Erection or Lubrication Problems	Impaired Orgasm	Hormonal Alteration*	Impotence
Adapin, Sinequan	Relief of depression	B		X	X	
Aldactazide, Aldactone	Control of high blood pressure; reduction of fluid retention	B			X	X
Aldoclor, Aldomet, Aldoril	Control of high blood pressure; reduction of fluid retention	B	X	X	X	X
Amicar	Treatment of excessive bleeding			X		
Antispasmodic capsules	Prevention of seizures			X		
Apresoline	Control of high blood pressure					X
Asendin	Relief of depression	B		X		X
Atromid-S	Lowering of cholesterol	B				X
Aventyl, Pamelor	Relief of depression	A or B				X
Bacarate	Suppression of appetite	A or B				X
Banthine	Relief of anxiety, insomnia; prevention of seizures					X
Bentyl	Control of irritable bowel					X
Cantil	Relief of ulcer pain					X
Catapres	Control of high blood pressure	B	X	X	X	X
Compazine	Control of psychoses, other mental disorders; relief of nausea, vomiting			X		
Dexedrine, other amphetamines	Treatment of narcolepsy; control of hyperactivity	B		X		X
Diamox	Control of glaucoma, convulsions; treatment of swelling	B				X
Dibenzyline	Control of high blood pressure			X		
Digoxin	Strengthening of heart muscle contractions	B				X
Dilantin	Prevention of seizures	B				
Diupres	Control of high blood pressure	B				X
Dolophine	Relief of pain	B		X		X
Donnatal	Relief of irritable bowel pain				X	X
Elavil, Endep, Triavil	Relief of depression	B		X	X	X
Esimil, Ismelin	Control of high blood pressure			X		X
Eskalith and other lithiums	Control of manic-depression					X
Estrogen drugs	Treatment of menstrual irregularities, menopause symptoms	B			X	
Eutonyl, Eutron	Control of high blood pressure			X		X
Haldol	Control of psychoses	A		X	X	X
Harmonyl, Moderil	Control of high blood pressure	B				X
Hydropres	Control of high blood pressure; reduction of fluid retention	B				X

*May include such diverse symptoms as breast enlargement and milk flow in both sexes; swelling of the testicles, reduced sperm count, change of voice pitch in men; menstrual irregularities, abnormal hairiness in women.

Possible Side Effects

Drug	Use	Increased (A) or Decreased (B) Sex Drive	Erection or Lubrication Problems	Impaired Orgasm	Hormonal Alteration*	Impotence
Hygroton	Control of high blood pressure; reduction of fluid retention	B				X
Inderal, Inderide	Reduction of angina; control of high blood pressure	B	X			X
Ionamin	Suppression of appetite	A or B				X
Librax	Relief of anxiety	A or B				
Librium	Relief of anxiety	A or B				
Lioresal	Relaxation of muscles					X
Lorelco	Lowering of cholesterol					X
Marplan	Relief of depression			X		X
Mellaril	Control of mental disorders		X	X	X	X
Minipress	Control of high blood pressure					X
Moban	Control of psychoses		X		X	
Naprosyn	Relief of inflammation			X		X
Nardil	Relief of depression			X		X
Navane	Control of psychoses			X	X	X
Neptazane	Treatment of glaucoma	B				X
Norlutin	Treatment of menstrual disorders	B				
Norpramin, Pertofrane	Relief of depression	B		X		X
Pamine	Relief of irritable bowel spasm		X			
Parnate	Relief of depression		X			X
Pathibamate	Relief of ulcer or irritable bowel pain					X
Phenobarbital, other barbiturates	Relief of anxiety, insomnia	B				
Pondimin	Suppression of appetite	B				X
Preludin	Suppression of appetite	A or B				X
Pro-Banthine	Relief of ulcer pain		X		X	X
Prolixin	Control of psychoses				X	X
Quide	Control of psychoses	A or B		X	X	
Rauzide	Control of high blood pressure	B				X
Ser-Ap-Es, Regroton, Sandril	Control of high blood pressure	B		X	X	X
Serentil	Treatment of psychoses		X	X		X
Serax	Relief of anxiety	B				
Stelazine	Control of psychoses		X	X		
Tagamet	Treatment of ulcers	B	X		X	X
Taractan	Treatment of psychoses			X	X	
Tenormin	Control of high blood pressure					X
Thorazine	Control of psychoses	B	X	X		X
Timoptic	Treatment of glaucoma	B				X
Tofranil	Relief of depression	B		X		X
Trecator-SC	Treatment of tuberculosis					X
Trilafon	Treatment of psychoses; control of severe nausea, vomiting			X	X	
Valium	Relief of anxiety	B		X		
Vivactil	Relief of depression	B			X	X

8

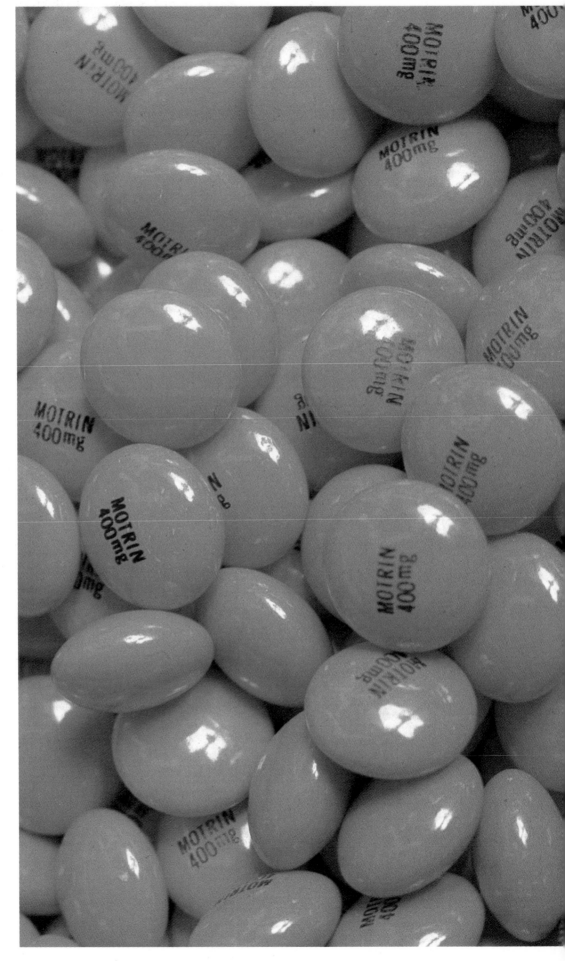

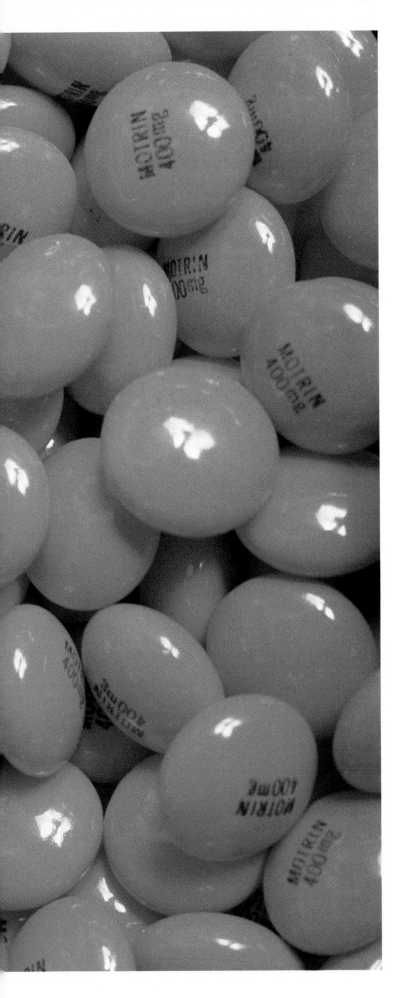

Commonly Prescribed Drugs

The prescription is in Latin; the drug seems mysteriously powerful. But you can learn about what you take.

There's a magic to medicine. Almost every culture in every age had a "medicine man" or some kind of healer with a special touch and a pouch full of secret ingredients to be consumed, smeared on, sprinkled in a certain way or just blown prayerfully to the four winds. In the face of illness, people gladly swallowed these sometimes-vile concoctions, smeared on the greasy unctions and generally submitted unquestioningly to the authority of this person who held their trust.

But that was in the past. Today, most people are savvy consumers of health care. They want to know more about medicines that have been prescribed for them—more than just how much to take and how often. They want to know what results they can expect from their medication. They want to be warned about side effects. They want to know if there are alternatives that may be less costly and less dangerous yet equally effective.

Certainly our doctors are willing to discuss the medications they prescribe. Yet often they are rushed. And sometimes they simply don't recognize that patients earnestly want this information and *can* understand it.

If you want to know more about a drug you are taking—or want to get the lowdown about what's likely to be prescribed for a suspected illness—turn to the alphabetical listing in this chapter of some of the most common diseases and health problems. Prescription drugs are listed under the conditions they are used for. Therefore, you will find a discussion of digitalis, for example, under the heading "Heart Disease" and information about Tagamet listed under "Digestive Disorders."

Information about these drugs comes straight from the experts, who evaluate the safety of a drug and tell you how it works.

121

Allergies and Asthma

Thirty-five million Americans suffer from allergies and asthma. Unlike infectious diseases, many of which science can prevent or swiftly cure with modern treatment, allergic symptoms can only be tempered and soothed.

The usual course of treatment is to first identify the allergen—that is, the substance causing the problem—and then, if at all possible, to avoid it. But when this simple preventive is not possible, doctors may suggest allergy "shots." This treatment stimulates a person's immunity to an allergen through injections of standard doses of the allergen itself, in steadily increasing quantities.

Allergy to Drugs

Allergic reactions to drugs occasionally can be serious. Asthma is one such reaction, and 1 out of 5 asthmatics has the most commonplace of all drugs to blame—aspirin. And if you're allergic to aspirin, studies show you're possibly sensitive to other substances that contain salicylates (the basis of aspirin). These include aspirinlike pain relievers—and several fruits. Moreover, those who are sensitive to aspirin also, for some unknown reason, react to FD&C Yellow No. 5 (tartrazine), which is used to color many drugs.

Another drug that can kick off an allergic reaction is penicillin, which may cause problems for up to 10 percent of the population. Flu shots (made from virus cultured on eggs) can cause a reaction in those who are *highly* allergic to eggs. Those diabetics who are allergic to beef and pork may want to try the nonanimal, genetically engineered forms of insulin.

In addition to drugs themselves, certain added colors, flavors or binders may generate problems.

Allergic people should learn all they can before they take any drug, whether it's prescribed by a doctor or purchased over the counter.

"SHOTS" FOR A FEW

It's sort of a "vaccination" against allergy, but it has its drawbacks. It can be done only with a select few allergies, and it does not promise complete protection. Sometimes it just doesn't work for certain people. Finally, the risk of triggering a full-blown allergic reaction during the injections is ever-present.

The next step may be to prescribe an allergy drug. Often that drug is an antihistamine such as Benadryl, Atarax or Vistaril.

This group of drugs is the jack-of-all-trades. Antihistamines dry up the stuffy nose of hay fever, relieve the itching of hives and quell the dizziness and queasy stomach of motion sickness, which can sometimes be symptoms of allergy.

Although they rarely have serious side effects, antihistamines may induce drowsiness, fatigue and confusion as well as loss of appetite, vomiting, abdominal pain and constipation or diarrhea. Their sedative effect warrants avoidance of alcoholic beverages and driving while taking antihistamines.

Nasal decongestant sprays and drops shrink swollen membranes in the nose and provide temporary relief of hay fever. Doctors are careful in prescribing decongestants, because they know that even the mildest may be habit forming. "The patient should only use them as needed," advises Frederic Speer, M.D., of Shawnee Mission, Kansas, "and get off them quickly if his nose is open only when he takes them."

TAKING STEROIDS

The most severe symptoms of allergies may be treated with steroid drugs—among them prednisone, prednisolone, dexamethasone, cortisone and hydrocortisone. In aerosol, pill and ointment form they treat all allergies, especially acute or chronic asthma, acute hives and drug reactions. Steroids suppress inflammation but their prolonged use also can suppress the body's ability to fight infection.

Doctors have found that risks can be minimized when steroids are taken in single morning doses during the body's own peak adrenal activity. Researchers have also found that high doses of vitamin C reversed cortisone's negative effect on the immune response. Salt restriction and potassium supplements can reduce the water retention. Taking steroids with a meal can counter their effects on the stomach. To limit effects on the skin, stay out of the sun if you are on steroids. And take vitamin D plus calcium supplements to reduce considerably the risk of broken bones.

Certain drugs are used specifically for asthma. One group is made up of bronchodilators, including ephedrine, epinephrine and theophylline. These are prescribed for asthmatics to relax the tightened bronchial muscles that block the free flow of air during an attack. The bronchodilator theophylline, related to caffeine, can have some severe side effects—anxiety, insomnia and tremor. Be careful in mixing coffee—or any product that contains caffeine—with theophylline. A UCLA research group conducted a study that concluded that the caffeine from as few as three cups of coffee can magnify the effect of theophylline on the central nervous system.

CATCHING YOUR BREATH

If exertion triggers asthma, as it does in nine out of ten cases, cromolyn sodium may be prescribed. This drug works by coating the cells of the membranes that line the lungs and bronchial tubes. It thus prevents the release of histamine, one of the body's chemical substances that raises havoc in the lungs during an allergic reaction.

None of these allergy and asthma drugs is anything to sneeze at. They're strong, but they're also necessary.

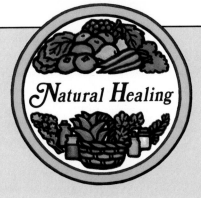

It's just common sense. Make every effort to control allergic conditions nonmedically first and minimize the need for drug therapy. In addition to avoiding the offending factors—foods, drugs, inhalants, country walks, animals—you can take some positive measures to bolster your defenses against allergy symptoms. There are several ways to do this.

- Vitamins A, B_6, C, and E all can help. Scientists at the National Cancer Institute showed that vitamin A can protect the lungs against the ravages of pollution. Vitamin B_6 relieved the wheezing and other symptoms in every asthmatic tested by a researcher with the U.S. Department of Agriculture. Vitamin C acts as a natural antihistamine, reducing the swelling and inflammation that cause discomfort in nasal and sinus tissues. Also, another study of vitamin C, this at Yale University, showed that when the vitamin was given, any bronchospasms experienced were much less severe. Vitamin E has also been shown effective in improving asthma symptoms.
- In addition to taking vitamin supplements, drink plenty of liquids (warm, not cold) to help thin mucus in the lungs so it can be coughed up. Warm liquids such as soup, herb tea or plain warm water also relax bronchial muscles.
- Studies have shown that moderate continuous physical activity can free congested nasal passages. Deep-breathing and warm-up exercises help asthmatics to handle exercise without stress.
- Acupuncture also seems to help asthma sufferers. Several Japanese researchers showed that acupuncture improved breathing significantly in asthmatic patients. Two studies reported in the *American Journal of Acupuncture* also concluded that acupuncture "has a very definite place in the treatment of asthma and could effectively eliminate asthma attacks for at least 6 months in 25 percent of the patients, while alleviating and minimizing symptoms in the large majority of patients treated."

Arthritis

The Kidney Punch

First the gastrointestinal tract. Now the kidneys. The latest target site for side effects from nonsteroidal anti-inflammatory drugs means another blow below the belt.

Basically two types of kidney-related abnormalities can occur, explains Allan B. Schwartz, M.D., a director of nephrology at Hahnemann University and Hospital, Philadelphia. "The first is an allergic reaction associated with acute kidney failure. The second, which occurs more frequently, involves a change in kidney function."

Swelling ankles, breathing difficulties, change in appetite, nausea, vomiting, lethargy and itching skin or rash are signals that a kidney malfunction may be developing.

What happens is that the NSAIDs do their job by suppressing the synthesis of a hormonal substance called prostaglandin. This substance is also important in regulating how the kidneys excrete sodium and protein. Thus, if the drug is effective against arthritis, some effect on the kidneys is anticipated.

"A lot of people who take NSAIDs get the swelling from salt and water retention, but it doesn't always lead to kidney failure." explains Jeffrey S. Stoff, M.D., from the department of medicine, University of Massachusetts. "People with congestive heart failure, previous kidney or liver disease, high blood pressure or lupus are at particularly high risk for the kidney problem," notes Dr. Stoff.

Both Dr. Stoff and Dr. Schwartz would discontinue use of NSAIDs in an individual if kidney problems arose, because the condition can be serious.

"These drugs should not be used without an examination of heart and kidneys and a urine test once a month from the start of the drugs," says Dr. Schwartz.

Arthritis sufferers, who often need medications just to get through the day, pay over a billion dollars a year and chance a litany of side effects. They are entitled to know whether the drugs' benefits outweigh their risks. Finding the answer means exploding a couple of myths.

Myth One: Arthritis medications are simple substances that just kill pain. Wrong. Antiarthritis agents are more than just painkillers. They actually work to cool inflammation.

Arthritis experts have drawn clear distinctions between such anti-inflammatories (including aspirin) and popular painkillers like Tylenol, Darvon and Demerol. In fact, most experts say that painkillers can do more harm than good.

Myth Two: An arthritis drug is equally effective for everyone with the same type of arthritis. Not so. The wide variations in the way people respond to arthritis medications are a matter of scientific record.

George Ehrlich, M.D., a rheumatologist and visiting professor of medicine at New York University School of Medicine, says, "People have to be patient, for a doctor may need to switch them from one medication to another to find one that's effective."

And the medicinal options are many. Here's a report card on the two most commonly prescribed categories.

The New Anti-Inflammatories. These chemically diverse substances sport brand names familiar to people with arthritis—Motrin, Indocin, Nalfon, Clinoril and others. Whatever type of arthritis yields to aspirin yields also to these nonsteroidal anti-inflammatory drugs (NSAIDs).

But the similarities stop there. For one thing, these drugs generally require less pill-taking to control rheumatoid arthritis (RA). Doctors and patients both know that the fewer pills you have to take, the more likely you are to take them.

And though NSAIDs cause most of the same side effects that aspirin does, the reactions are generally less severe. Some doctors, however, caution that it's too early to hail NSAIDs as safer alternatives to aspirin. "Aspirin has been used for centuries," says James F. Fries, M.D., director of the Stanford University Arthritis Clinic, "whereas experience with these new drugs is sufficiently limited that some side effects may not yet have been discovered."

Then there are those few NSAIDs that are giving the others a bad name. Oraflex and Zomax were removed from the market in 1984 because they were associated with deaths. And the serious side effects caused by phenylbutazone (Butazolidin) and indomethacin (Indocin) have raised grave doubts about their use.

An American Medical Association (AMA) guide to medications says that phenylbutazone can cause jaundice, hepatitis, blood in the urine, edema, rashes, gastrointestinal disturbances and—worst of all—a dangerous form of bone marrow toxicity.

Indocin shares many of phenylbutazone's possible side effects (including bone marrow toxicity) and has some bizarre reactions of its own: eye disturbances, kidney trouble, confusion, coma, even behavioral problems. Perhaps most worrisome of all are the possible ulcerations of the esophagus, stomach and small intestine, which, the AMA says, are sometimes fatal.

The Steroids. In the 1950s these substances took the medical world by storm. Cortisone—the first of the steroid drugs—actually enabled RA cripples to walk, run and even jump, free of pain. But then reality set in. It soon became clear that a dose of cortisone strong enough to suppress the disease could produce an alarming range of toxic effects, from the unsightly "moon face" to perforating and bleeding gastric ulcers. And now, 30 years after the steroid

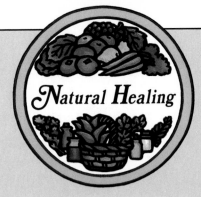

Natural Healing

In conjunction with your medication, some natural methods also can help your arthritis. Certain conditions seem to respond to nutritional supplements, a low-fat diet and the right exercise. So consider some of the following findings when planning your own three-pronged attack.
- An Israeli study showed that vitamin E provides marked relief from pain in osteoarthritis.
- A study done in Denmark found that people with psoriatic arthritis improved significantly when they took zinc supplements.
- Cod-liver oil supplements helped relieve fatigue, swelling and immobility, according to a study done at Brusch Medical Center in Cambridge, Massachusetts.
- Exercises like swimming, stretching and walking help increase flexibility and relieve pain.
- A low-fat diet seems to eliminate the pain and stiffness of RA, say 2 doctors at Wayne State University in Detroit.

debut, doctors are still wielding this medicinal two-edged sword—but more gingerly.

A BALANCING ACT

Nowadays doctors walk the thin line between this positive force and side effects like ulcers, skin disorders, bone disease and cataracts. And they do this by carefully controlling dosages and duration of treatment.

Weighing risks against benefits is the arthritis sufferer's lot—a serious business that requires a respect for medicinal power and a need for straight answers.

Cancer

When German bombs fell on a convoy of Allied ships in Italy during World War II, not a soul could have guessed that such brutal destruction would catalyze the discovery of a healing agent for a killer disease. The men on the ships were accidentally exposed to poisonous mustard gas which, autopsies later suggested, contained an element that might be active against cancer cells. The mustard compounds that eventually resulted from follow-up research were among the first cancer-killing drugs and are still used today.

Chemotherapy, the use of drugs or chemicals to treat diseases such as cancer, is still a relatively new field. Thirty years ago there were not even oncologists—doctors who specialize in treating this country's second leading killer. Now chemotherapy, with 45 to 50 compounds in use, heralds a new age of improving survival rates for many types of cancer, as researchers test thousands of drugs, approving 1 in every 15,000.

"We've almost conquered leukemia," is the succinct belief of one doctor at the National Cancer Institute (NCI) in Washington, D.C. That conquest began in 1949 with the discovery of methotrexate, which was found effective against leukemia in children as well as against choriocarcinoma, a rare cancer of the fetal membrane the once killed five out of six of its victims within a year. Today more than half the children who contract leukemia survive at least five years, after which time the chance of relapse is one in ten. And about three-fourths of the women afflicted with choriocarcinoma experience complete remission.

Following on the heels of these crucial breakthroughs is a growing list of drugs that have significantly raised the survival and cure rates for other types of cancer. The new generation of chemotherapy drugs is used more and more to enhance the effectiveness of surgery and radiation, formerly the big guns. Because drugs reach all tissues, chemotherapy holds more hope of response from cancers that infest the whole body, such as cancer of the blood or lymph system.

Chemotherapy may also be used for reaching microscopic cancer cells that elude surgery and radiation. Cytoxan, methotrexate and 5-fluorouracil are drugs that have been shown successful in preventing recurrences of breast cancer.

BATTLING SIDE EFFECTS

Like many medical treatments, chemotherapy offers a bittersweet mixture of hope and dread. It prompts the hope of survival, which helps those stricken with cancer to face the sometimes (though not always) dreadful side effects of chemotherapy. These reactions include nausea, vomiting, hair loss, fatigue, mouth sores and sterility, as well as severe toxic effects to blood-forming cells and the heart and kidneys. The treatment may also lead to the development of new cancers.

Not all cancer drugs cause the same spectrum of side effects, and tolerance and reactions vary widely, often depending on the individual. Fortunately, there are antidotes to counter some of the unpleasant side effects such as nausea. One of the most effective is a direct descendant of the 1960s drug culture. THC (tetrahydrocannabinol), the active ingredient in marijuana, counters nausea and acts as a sedative and appetite stimulant. Since 1980 the NCI has been authorized to distribute a form of THC, and many hospitals now have access to it. In addition, several prescription drugs called antiemetics also help to control nausea. These include Compazine and metoclopramide.

All cancer drugs are toxic and work by interrupting some vital stage of cell division. Most cancer cells are vulnerable to a drug's effect when they are dividing, which they do very rapidly. The main drawback of these drugs is that they destroy not only dividing cancer cells but also normal cells that divide rapidly. These normal cells are found in the stomach and intestines, mucus membranes, hair follicles and bone marrow—hence the notorious side effects at these sites.

Chemotherapy Self-Care

When Grace Becker, a 29-year-old nurse, was told she would have to receive chemotherapy, she had a very *human* reaction—in the face of cancer, she worried about becoming bald. Fortunately, she did not experience this common side effect of cancer therapy. And, putting her nursing experience to good use on herself, she worked hard to counter other unwanted effects. In fact, she developed a program of self-care that not only helped physically but also allowed Grace "to feel some sense of control" over the chemotherapy treatment.

Although doctors told Grace she'd be on the drugs for about a year, her condition responded to the treatment in only 2 months. Three months after starting chemotherapy, Grace felt so good she ran her first marathon in Boston.

According to a report in *American Medical News,* scientific evidence shows that the side effects of chemotherapy can be lessened by nonmedical procedures such as hypnosis, biofeedback, sequential muscle tensing and relaxing and guided imagery to achieve deep muscle relaxation.

In addition to counseling and relaxation techniques, you also can develop an effective home care regimen. Because chemotherapy kills not only cancer cells but also other cells that reproduce rapidly, side effects usually occur in specific areas of the body—the mouth, the digestive tract, the hair follicles. Marylin Dodd, R.N., Ph.D., a professor of nursing at the University of California, San Francisco, has found simple, effective measures you can use at home to prevent or limit these side effects. In her comprehensive manual, *Suggestions for Managing the Side Effects of Chemo-therapy,* Dr. Dodd suggests treating nausea with remedies "we all grew up with—drinking 7-Up, taking a nap, going on a clear-liquid diet, eating crackers, taking over-the-counter drugs." Her 123-page manual also includes 44 possible chemotherapy side effects and takes the time (which many doctors simply don't have) to spell out self-care measures.

To reduce the common side effect of mouth sores, Dr. Dodd recommends these measures:

- Drink plenty of liquids to keep your mouth moist.
- Brush your teeth with a baby-soft toothbrush.
- Cleanse dentures after every meal to remove irritating food particles and to help prevent infection.
- Floss your teeth daily, but very gently. Or use a WaterPik at a low setting.
- Avoid very hot or very cold foods.
- Make your own nonirritating mouth rinse by mixing 1 teaspoon of baking soda with 1 cup of warm water. Keep this rinse in your mouth for about 1 minute and repeat every 4 hours while awake.
- Apply a lubricant such as Vaseline to your lips to keep them moist.
- Eat bland and cool soft foods such as custards, yogurt, soups and eggs. Avoid foods such as oranges, tomatoes, lemons, limes, raw vegetables or heavily spiced foods, since they may irritate your mouth.
- If your home is heated by dry heat, a humidifier may help.
- Avoid cigarettes and alcohol.

Dr. Dodd advises people receiving chemotherapy to tell their doctors about all side effects to help them decide if the reactions are normal or if a dosage should be modified.

Rarely does a single drug cure a malignancy. Instead, combinations are used to ensure 100 percent eradication of the cancer. Leaving even .001 percent of the cancer cells will result in a regrowth of the malignancy.

It makes sense for the cancer patient to become familiar with the triumphs and failures of chemotherapy, for the effectiveness of drugs may change rapidly as new strides in cancer research are made.

Diabetes

Not many people think of insulin when miracle drugs are discussed, but before its discovery in 1921, developing diabetes was virtually a death sentence. With this drug, people stricken with a once-fatal disease can lead normal and active lives.

And not many people expect an effective treatment for America's third leading cause of death to be an over-the-counter drug. But it is, and each year some of the 3 percent of all Americans who are diagnosed diabetics may be thankful for it.

Diabetes is a condition that leads to excessive amounts of sugar (in the metabolized form of glucose) in the blood. About 15 percent of all diabetics have what is known as Type I diabetes. Also called juvenile-onset or insulin-dependent diabetes, it is believed to be hereditary. With this disease, the pancreas fails to produce adequate amounts of insulin, a hormone that helps the body's cells utilize glucose. For people with Type I, daily insulin injections are indispensable.

Frequent blood sugar checks are the best indicator of an individual's exact need for insulin. When blood sugar is high, the insulin level should be high. When the blood sugar level is low, the insulin level should be low.

"Patients should monitor their own blood sugar," says Stanley Mirsky, M.D., associate clinical professor of metabolic diseases at Mt. Sinai School of Medicine, City College, New York. "Insulin dosage is a very individual thing and it needs to be checked frequently. The doctor determines with the patient how to best distribute the insulin. Most of my patients have their own glucose-monitoring system."

"It's also important to take insulin in a consistent manner based on instructions from a doctor," says Daniel Porte, M.D., director of diabetes research at the University of Washington. Different kinds of insulin work for different lengths of time. Fast-acting insulin starts to work in about ½ hour, has its peak effect in 2 to 3 hours and lasts about 6 hours. Slow-acting insulin, called NPH and lente, starts working about 2 to 3 hours after injection, peaks in 8 to 16 hours and has a duration of about 24 hours. An individual's constitution and lifestyle can influence which type is prescribed. But whatever type a person uses, it's important to realize there's no such thing as "generic" insulin.

"One thing diabetics should know," says Dr. Porte, "is that brands of insulin are made differently and are not identical. They have different degrees of purity. Unless specifically directed, diabetics should not switch brands. Also, sometimes there are

Monitoring Insulin

"Patients can learn to adjust their own insulin dosage—it's very easy," says John N. Douglass, M.D., of Los Angeles. "The old method," says Dr. Douglass, "was to check the urine 3 to 4 times a day. Now there is a blood test. You prick yourself and monitor blood sugar with a sort of dipstick by comparing the color of the dipstick with the color on a chart. Usually once a day is enough."

Monitoring your blood sugar will help you figure out when your insulin is having its strongest effect, so your doctor can prescribe a dosage schedule that will use up the right amount of sugar after you eat. Carefully recording the results of blood sugar tests is the most efficient way to help control diabetes.

The newest device for helping diabetics monitor and record blood sugar is a miniature insulin dosage computer, about the size of a pocket calculator. The battery-powered device dispenses insulin dosage advice based on information the patient punches into it.

Its inventor says that many patients—young diabetics, in particular—develop a fondness for their "little friend" that greets them by name, plays tunes and politely asks particulars about their upcoming meal, latest blood sugar levels, the day, date and so forth. The machine processes this information, then flashes instructions on its tiny screen, with recommendations for the insulin dosage.

specials on different brands in pharmacies. The diabetic should be careful before buying these and check with the doctor first."

Allergic reactions to insulin are not uncommon in the first few weeks of treatment. Reactions can be local (redness, swelling and itching) or generalized (rashes, breathing difficulty, rapid pulse and low blood pressure). Notify your doctor if any of these problems arise. Sometimes switching insulin alleviates the problem. Most insulin comes from the pancreas of both cows and pigs, but pure pork insulin has a chemical composition closest to human insulin and is less likely to cause side effects.

A highly purified type of insulin called monocomponent also is less likely to cause reactions at injection sites. In some cases, human insulin may be recommended. Be warned: It's very expensive.

Store insulin that you use daily at room temperature and store the rest of it in the refrigerator. Never keep any insulin past its expiration date.

When using their insulin, "diabetics should rotate the site of injection," says John N. Douglass, M.D., a Los Angeles internist. This general practice helps avoid scarring or lumping in any one area, a problem that can affect the absorption of insulin. Thighs, buttocks, abdomen and upper parts of the arm—which all have substantial fat pads—are the usual sites for the subcutaneous (beneath the skin) injections.

For the 11 million Americans who suffer from Type II (maturity-onset) diabetes, a lack of insulin is not necessarily their problem. In fact, their insulin levels may even be higher than normal, but the hormone is delinquent in performing its duties.

A low-fat, high-fiber diet (one rich in complex carbohydrates) is the treatment of choice recommended by the American Diabetes Association and the British Diabetic Association since 1979 for Type II diabetics. For others, weight loss has brought a total disappearance of the disease. Exercise, too, has been shown to be

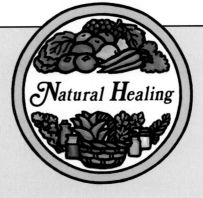

Natural Healing

Natural control of diabetes begins with two big don'ts: DON'T eat foods high in refined sugar and DON'T eat lots of fats, especially saturated fats. Refined sugar enters the bloodstream quickly, increasing sugar levels rapidly and causing a large surge of insulin. Eventually your body needs larger-than-normal amounts of insulin to do a normal job. When fat enters the bloodstream it interferes with insulin's action, preventing it from lowering your blood sugar.

Among other natural means of control for diabetes are two dos: DO eat meals rich in fiber. They help insulin function normally and even lessen the need for it. DO make sure your diet includes linoleic acid, an essential fatty acid that is found in sunflower and safflower oils and is useful in fighting the deadly circulatory side effects of diabetes.

important. It helps restore normal metabolism and enhances the action of insulin.

In addition to dietary treatment, Type II diabetics may take oral drugs instead of insulin injections. The most common pills are called sulfonylureas. They help the pancreas release enough insulin to normalize the blood sugar and they help the insulin do its job throughout the body. Some of the side effects of antidiabetes pills include dark urine, unusual tiredness, fever, sore throat, unusual bleeding, bruising and yellowing of the whites of the eyes.

In 1979 a research review confirmed a controversial finding first published in 1970 that diabetics who take oral drugs to lower their blood sugar may have an increased risk of fatal heart attack. But the good news is that no diabetic need undergo such risks. Diabetes is one of the most controllable diseases with proper diet and exercise. Ask your doctor about such a program.

Digestive Disorders _____

Although exact causes are known for only a few digestive ailments, many successful treatments are available.

Take the case of ulcers. Since 1977 the FDA has approved three new prescription drugs for ulcers—cimetidine (Tagamet), ranitidine (Zantac) and sucralfate (Carafate)—and all have very good safety profiles.

These drugs relieve ulcer pain and reduce the corrosive effect of acid and pepsin, powerful digestive juices that can burn the lining of the stomach and duodenum, the first part of the intestine. (Those are the two sites of ulcers: gastric in the stomach; duodenal in the duodenum.)

"Cimetidine and ranitidine essentially work by preventing secretion of acid in the stomach," says Gail L. Bongiovanni, M.D., assistant professor of clinical medicine at the University of Cincinnati College of Medicine. "Antacids buffer the acid, but these two drugs actually prevent acid from being produced."

Of the two, ranitidine seems better. Although eight times more potent, it usually has less serious side effects than cimetidine, says Arnold G. Levy, M.D., associate clinical professor of medicine at George Washington University Medical Center and vice president for educational affairs, American Digestive Disease Society. Cimetidine may cause mental confusion in the elderly or in people with impaired kidney function. Moreover, it may also cause drug interactions, says Dr. Bongiovanni. "Ranitidine has fewer drug interactions—that's one of its major advantages," she continues. "Cimetidine can have very potent antiandrogen effects. It can feminize men, making them impotent and causing their breasts to develop. Ranitidine almost never does that."

BAND-AID DRUG

Sucralfate, a drug completely different from cimetidine and ranitidine, is presently approved only for duodenal ulcers. "It basically works by adhering to areas of the stomach or the duodenal lining that have lost their cover or have been ulcerated," says Dr. Levy. "It's almost as if you put a protective coating over the ulcer. But since it's only a chemical barrier, it has essentially no buffering capacity. So it does not really absorb acid."

Because your system absorbs only about 5 percent of sucralfate, the incidence of side effects is low and they are relatively minor. Its major side effect is constipation in a small percentage of those who use it. However, when it is taken with cimetidine, both drugs are less effective.

If you smoke and take any of these drugs for an ulcer, be warned that smoking may undermine the drug's effects. "Studies have shown that ulcer patients who take drugs for their condition and smoke have a higher incidence of relapse than those who take the drugs and don't smoke," says Lawrence S. Friedman, M.D., assistant professor of medicine, Thomas Jefferson University, Philadelphia.

IRRITABLE INSIDES

One of the most common digestive disorders, irritable bowel syndrome (IBS), results from a disturbance of the bowel's normal pattern of contraction. It can cause chronic diarrhea, constipation and abdominal pain. Some relief can be gained from a group of drugs called anticholinergics or antispasmodics, including Bentyl, Donnatal and Librax. These drugs relax the bowel wall and control the painful spasms of IBS.

Before recommending these drugs, Dr. Levy treats IBS with a high-fiber diet, fiber supplements or both. He also eliminates known irritants such as caffeine and fried or fatty foods.

Much more serious than IBS is inflammatory bowel disease (IBD). Flare-ups are quite debilitating and inflame the bowel wall.

"There are basically two types of IBD," says Dr. Levy. "One is ulcerative colitis, which is an inflammatory process in the lining of the colon. The other is Crohn's disease, an inflammatory process that affects all of the bowel wall from the inside lining to the outside covering and involves both small and large intestines.''

Many people with ulcerative colitis can control it by taking sulfasalazine (Azulfidine). This drug is metabolized by intestinal bacteria into two parts, one of which is an aspirinlike compound. "It's the aspirinlike part that does the job," says Dr. Bongiovanni, but it's not clear how it works. Plain aspirin isn't effective, she adds.

What is clear, though, is that the drug can have side effects. The most usual are allergy to the drug or upset stomach. According to Dr. Bongiovanni, an upset stomach usually can be avoided by gradually increasing doses, rather than starting out with maximum doses.

Dr. Bongiovanni advises people on Azulfidine to take a folate supplement. Although this vitamin is found abundantly in orange juice, liver, romaine lettuce and beets, the drug interferes with its metabolism.

Prednisone, a more potent anti-inflammatory agent, is a steroid drug usually given in more severe cases of IBD. "Mild cases of ulcerative colitis may be treatable with just Azulfidine," says Dr. Bongiovanni.

A drug used to treat extreme cases of Crohn's disease is azathioprine, which is converted by the liver into something called 6-mercaptopurine (6-MP). This substance, an anticancer drug, is prednisone-sparing (that is, doctors sometimes prescribe it not only as an anti-inflammatory, but also to decrease the dose requirement of prednisone). "However," says Dr. Levy, "it may have a cancer-*producing* effect 20 or 30 years down the road, so the situation has to be pretty advanced before it's used." As with other cancer-related drugs, 6-MP's greatest potential harm is to the bone marrow. "But most people tolerate the drug in the doses that are commonly used," says Dr. Levy.

ALTERNATIVE TO SURGERY

The drug chenodiol (Chenix) is prescribed to dissolve gallstones.

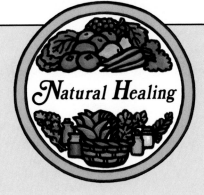

Natural Healing

You can help prevent—or heal—the digestive problems discussed on these 2 pages by paying attention to what you digest. First on that list is fiber, the food factor that helps keep bowel movements normal. Research shows that fiber can help prevent ulcers and gallstones, as well as other digestive problems not discussed here, like hiatal hernia, colon cancer, diverticulosis and appendicitis. A totally fiberless food—sugar—has been linked to the development of Crohn's disease and irritable bowel syndrome. And a diet overloaded with fat (which also has no fiber) plays a role in gallstones.

What you drink can be just as important as what you eat: A glass of water before and after meals may help soothe ulcers, according to one doctor. So might a diet rich in vitamin A foods, like green and yellow vegetables. Vitamin A is also important for people with Crohn's disease, who may also need extra amounts of zinc, which can help control some of the symptoms of the problem.

(Prescriptions are limited, however, to those who are too old or too ill to withstand surgery, which is the usual treatment.) This digestive problem causes about 500,000 Americans each year to give up their gallbladders to a surgeon. Gallstones develop when excess cholesterol forms into stonelike crystals. When they cause obstruction or severe local irritation they can cause piercing pain. Surgery has been the traditional treatment when the obstruction or inflammation does not subside. Chenodiol will dissolve cholesterol gallstones *if* they are small and "floating" (not heavy or dense enough to sink in the bile, the liquid substance contained in the gallbladder). Taken over 6 to 12 months, it works in about 70 percent of all cases. Stones, however, will re-form once the drug is stopped. The drug has some side effects— diarrhea and the possibility of liver damage.

Eye Disease

Janet had been a safe, accident-free driver for 30 years, so the crash really shook her up. Her vision was fine without glasses, and her eyes never bothered her. So why didn't she see the car that slammed into her from the right?

Because Janet has glaucoma, an eye condition that strikes 1 person in 50 over the age of 35 and affects blacks ten times as often as whites. Glaucoma tends to run in families, and the chances of getting it increase as you get older.

There are two main types of glaucoma, open-angle, which Janet and at least 90 percent of glaucoma victims have, and closed-angle. Open-angle glaucoma is called the "silent thief" of sight because its victims may not notice gradual, painless symptoms like progressive loss of side vision until it's too late. Closed-angle glaucoma announces itself with sharp, sudden eye and head pains. Left untreated, they both can cause blindness.

Both types of glaucoma are caused when fluid in the eyeball, which normally drains away, builds up. The pressure inside the eyeball rises as the fluid increases, gradually destroying the optic nerve.

TIMOPTIC: PROS AND CONS

That's where glaucoma drugs come in. The newest and best of these is Timoptic, the first new glaucoma drug in 25 years. It lowers the pressure inside the eye, with fewer side effects than older glaucoma drugs.

"Timoptic is nearly always the first drug of choice against glaucoma," says Jimmy D. Bartlett, O.D., associate professor of optometry at the University of Alabama School of Optometry. "It's used 60 to 70 percent of the time, but the occurrence of side effects can run as high as 10 percent of all patients," he says.

Why? Because Timoptic is a beta blocker that—in addition to its glaucoma use—can lower blood pressure. Timoptic is absorbed into the bloodstream through the eyes, and if you have severe asthma or heart problems, it could trigger respiratory failure or a heart attack.

And if you're already on a beta blocker (for high blood pressure) and you start taking Timoptic for glaucoma, you could be putting yourself in double jeopardy. The combined effect can lower the action of your heart and lungs to a dangerous crawl.

Don't assume the eye doctor who prescribes a new medication

How to Apply Eye Medication

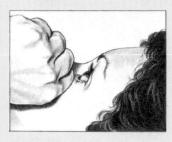

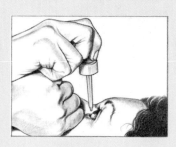

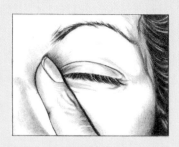

Ophthalmologist Joseph M. Ortiz, M.D., tells a story about a patient who complained her eye medication wasn't working. Asked to demonstrate how she applied her eye drops, she filled a paper cup half full and threw it in her eyes.

Considering the cost of eye medication, that's more tragic than comic. To apply eye drops safely and painlessly, says Dr. Ortiz, first tilt your head back so it's parallel to the floor. Now make your left hand into a fist if you're right-handed (right hand if you're a southpaw), and put it under the lower eyelid, gently pulling down.

Take the filled eye-dropper in your right hand (vice versa for lefties), rest your right hand on your left fist and drop the medication into the lower eyelid. Now press your index finger to the corner of your eye closest to your nose and hold it there for 10 seconds with your eye closed. Reverse hands and repeat for the other eye.

To apply salve, squeeze about an inch gently into your lower eyelid, with your hands in the position described previously.

knows what other medications you're taking. Telling him could save both of you an awful lot of trouble.

OLDIES, NOT GOODIES

For glaucoma patients who can't take Timoptic, ophthalmologists prescribe older drugs like epinephrine and pilocarpine. But these drugs have many more annoying side effects than Timoptic. They can make your eyes sting and turn bright red and give you hammering headaches. Not surprisingly, many people won't take them.

ZAPPING GLAUCOMA

The latest glaucoma research has much more of light touch than drug therapy: lasers.

The word conjures up images of space saga derring-do, but some researchers claim high-tech laser surgery will one day replace all existing glaucoma drugs. Right now, it may be no more permanent than drug therapy and must be performed repeatedly.

Patients frequently have to stay on glaucoma drugs like Timoptic both before and after the procedure anyway. Says Dr. Bartlett, "It's new and impressive, but so far it's just an adjunct to drug therapy in most cases."

GETTING THE RED OUT

Back here on planet Earth, most of us never get glaucoma or have laser beams pointed at our eyes. But everyone occasionally gets smarting, sore, scratchy eyes that scream for relief. The specks of dirt, fungi, bacteria and viruses that blow into our eyes from who knows where can cause eye infections. The most common is conjunctivitis, or "pinkeye," a bacterial infection. This kind of infection isn't too serious. But what seems like really bad news is the stream of puslike stuff that oozes out of your eyes. That symptom will probably send you to your doctor in a hurry. Once you're there—and

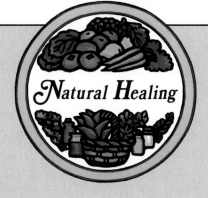

Natural Healing

Bugs Bunny can see very well what's up, even without a doctor. Bugs, after all, eats lots of vitamin A-rich carrots. It's true that a deficiency of vitamin A is one of the causes of glaucoma, but there's more to the picture than that.

Several eye researchers have noticed that vitamin C seems to lower eye pressure. Joseph Ortiz, M.D., recommends vitamin C to all his patients, and says the pressure may sometimes be reduced by taking as little as 250 milligrams a day, under a physician's guidance.

And to clear up conjunctivitis, a Dutch researcher found that vitamin B_6 might help. Microorganisms that cause pinkeye lived 30 to 37 percent longer in the eyes of B_6-deficient animals. And Dr. Ortiz reports vitamin C and zinc aspartate dissolved under the tongue also help.

reassured you're not about to go blind—the doctor will usually prescribe an antibiotic like tobramycin, gentamycin or sulfacetamide, all of which are safe. Only one, Neosporin, has frequent side effects, and they are usually limited to allergic reactions like redness, itching and stinging.

STEROIDS: NOT FOR THE EYE

Be sure to ask which drug is being prescribed, not only to make sure you're getting the safest antibiotic but also to be sure you're *not* getting a steroid. These are often prescribed for eye infections, and they can have severe side effects. They do reduce the inflammation faster than antibiotics but unlike antibiotics, they do nothing to fight infection.

Steroid eye drops may also *cause* devastating conditions like glaucoma and cataracts. Diabetics and people with glaucoma and myopia (nearsightedness) are particularly at risk, says one doctor, writing in the *Western Journal of Medicine*.

Heart Disease

In the year 1984 heart surgeons attempted to prolong the life of an infant girl by implanting in her the heart of a baboon. That same year two other diseased human hearts were completely replaced with artificial devices. Not many of the estimated 40 million sufferers of this nation's leading killer expect to be treated with such dramatic measures. Instead, many of those with heart disease are treated with a variety of drugs.

Digitalis, for example, has long been used to treat congestive heart failure. In 1785 the English physician William Withering learned of the remedy from a folk healer who used foxglove (a common garden flower) to reduce fluid retention. Dr. Withering extracted the herb's active substance and today, 200 years later, we still use the drug.

Congestive heart failure is a condition in which the heart's pumping action is impaired. The heart becomes enlarged, the kidneys retain salt and water and fluids can backwash into the lungs, causing shortness of breath. Digitalis helps both to increase the strength of the heart's contractions and to reduce the heart to about normal size. The drug is also used to treat a heart that's beating too quickly. In this case, the drug slows the heart so it doesn't work as hard. At the same time it increases the force of the heart's contraction so it gets more "beat for its buck," so to speak.

Your doctor will, no doubt, monitor you very closely if you are on digitalis to see if you display signs of sensitivity. This drug's chief drawback is that it may accumulate in the body in amounts that can be poisonous.

Digitalis also can interact with some over-the-counter drugs and allergy and cold remedies that contain antihistamines, so be sure to inform your doctor of all medication you're on.

Vasodilators are another class of drugs that counter the symptoms of hypertension (high blood pressure) or congestive heart failure. As their name implies, they dilate, or open up, the arteries or veins, decreasing the resistance against which the weakened heart must pump. They also can help reduce the volume of blood circulating in the lungs that contributes to the shortness of breath associated with a failing heart.

Again, different drugs in this class act differently. For example, the drugs hydralazine and diazoxide primarily open up arterioles (the smallest arteries), while nitroprusside and prazosin dilate both arterioles and veins.

Diuretics are yet another group of drugs used to treat a symptom of congestive heart failure. They help the kidneys eliminate excess sodium and water.

RELIEVING ANGINA

Beta blockers are a class of drugs used to treat angina pectoris, chest pains that occur when the heart requires more oxygen than clogged arteries can supply. The beta blockers help to prevent this frightening condition by slowing down the heart's rate of contraction. When you decrease the heart's speed, you also lower its demand for oxygen. Propanolol (Inderal) is one of the most common beta blockers used for angina.

Doctors may sometimes advise heart patients to keep handy a drug

New Nitro Treatment

People with angina or severe coronary disease can absorb their daily dose of nitroglycerin from an inconspicuous, half-dollar-sized patch that they apply themselves to any part of their bodies. Usually the patch (called Nitrodisc, Transderm or Nitro-Dur) is worn alternately on the upper left or right arm or the upper chest, and it does not interfere with swimming or showering.

Unlike oral nitrates, which must be administered several times a day, the patch works for 24 hours. Although its side effects are less marked, you may still experience some of the headaches and dizziness associated with taking nitroglycerin.

called nitroglycerin to relieve the pain of angina. Nitroglycerin decreases the workload on the heart by decreasing the resistance of blood flowing from the heart in the arteries and reducing the amount of blood returned to the heart by the veins.

ABNORMAL BEATS

Arrhythmia, a condition where the heart's beating rate falls outside the normal range of 60 to 100 lub-dubs per minute, can be corrected with any of a group of drugs aptly named antiarrhythmics. To properly select the best drug for you, your doctor must take into account several factors, including your tolerance, any diseases you may have and whether or not you smoke. Next, he determines which part of the heart is affected. For example, a drug called quinidine is usually prescribed for an arrhythmia in the atrial muscle (the upper part of the heart) and one called lidocaine is prescribed when the ventricular muscle (the lower part) is affected.

UNJAMMING THE LIFELINE

A lifetime of eating well—marbled beef, deep-fried foods and other dishes high in fat and cholesterol—can contribute to a disease known as atherosclerosis. Atherosclerosis not only leads to hypertension but also can cause a heart attack.

The arteries, the lifeline of blood, become more jammed than a New York subway at rush hour. Their walls are lined with a buildup of plaque (a sludge of fats). People with atherosclerosis may develop blood clots. To lessen the likelihood of this danger, doctors may prescribe anticoagulants to keep clots from forming. The two most common drugs of this sort are warfarin and bishydroxycoumarin.

Both these drugs have a potentially troublesome side effect—they interfere with the body's ability to use vitamin K, a substance necessary for normal blood clotting. This interference sometimes can result in serious internal or external bleeding.

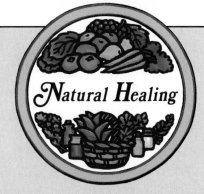

Natural Healing

You're already winning the battle the natural way! "The death rate from heart disease is down 35 percent in the past 15 years." says Adrian Ostfeld, M.D., professor of epidemiology and public health at Yale University School of Medicine, who attributes this significant victory largely to healthy lifestyle changes and improved detection and treatment of high blood pressure. "Twenty-five million Americans have stopped smoking since 1964," says Dr. Ostfeld, and that's a big step toward snuffing out the risk of heart disease.

Another heartening change is Americans' changed dietary habits: eating less animal fat and fewer eggs, and replacing whole milk with skim. Add to these creditable habits America's growing passion for jogging and leisure exercise and you have a nation on the right track to a healthy heart.

Therefore, doctors may advise patients to carry vitamin K tablets, which they can take at the first sign of any serious bleeding. Frequent supervision is necessary while you are on these drugs.

Because aspirin also can decrease platelet aggregation—which can further slow clotting time—it's probably wise to avoid taking it with anticoagulants.

All heart drugs have some side effects. One doctor explains the risk this way: "The risk of taking heart drugs is roughly equal to the risk of crossing a busy intersection." Side effects range from the headache, rash, dizziness and sexual dysfunction associated with some drugs used in the treatment of high blood pressure and heart attack to the possible mental effects of digitalis and related drugs.

Doctors can minimize all these adverse effects by finding the right drug to accommodate each individual's tolerance and by monitoring the patient throughout treatment.

High Blood Pressure

Chances are that someone you know—maybe even you—suffers from high blood pressure. And chances are that it's being treated with some type of medication. While diet, relaxation and weight control all play an important role in keeping blood pressure at the right level, drugs are still the most common treatment. They are common because even though all blood pressure drugs have side effects, they work well for treating this serious disease.

And serious it is. High blood pressure (hypertension) is directly tied to heart attacks and strokes. If you are among the 60 million Americans with a blood pressure problem and are between the ages of 45 and 74, you are three times as likely to have a heart attack and seven times as likely to have a stroke as someone with normal blood pressure. An estimated 850,000 people die each year from hypertension-related heart diseases.

DRUGS SAVE LIVES

Given these facts, antihypertensive drugs are "lifesavers in that they prevent the long-term complications that come with high blood pressure," says Norman M. Kaplan, M.D., head of the hypertension section at the University of Texas Southwestern Medical School in Dallas.

This view is echoed by Herbert Langford, M.D., of the University of Mississippi Medical School in Jackson. "All of the blood pressure medications have serious side effects. However, the benefits outweigh the risks. The drugs work," he says.

There are three main types of drugs—diuretics, sympathetic nervous inhibitors and vasodilators—that all achieve the same result: lowered pressure. High blood pressure occurs when blood vessels are overfilled and tight, like a thin hose hooked to a strong faucet. The diuretics increase the body's output of urine by taking some of the fluid and sodium from your blood vessels, making them less tight. The vasodilators act directly on the blood vessel to dilate it, much the same as you would loosen a belt after a big meal. The sympathetic inhibitors, including beta blockers, cause the nerves surrounding the blood vessel to stop the flow of adrenaline, thereby widening the vessels. All three drugs cause the pressure to drop and the blood to flow more easily.

All three can also cause serious side effects, including dizziness, stomach upset, ulcers, depression, diarrhea, dry mouth, sexual dysfunction, slowed heart rate, cough and potassium depletion. Still, because there are so many different types of antihypertension drugs available, there is no real reason why anyone should suffer any especially unpleasant side effects.

The fact is that all three categories of drugs work differently in

---

Drugs for High Blood Pressure —Maybe Not for Life

"Once on diuretics, always on diuretics." This adage of doctors who believe high blood pressure drugs (of which fluid-draining diuretics are one type) must be taken for life may be false, according to a study done at the University of Toronto.

Martin G. Meyers, M.D., and his associates switched a group of diuretic-taking elderly people with high blood pressure to a placebo. Another, similar group continued taking diuretics. Neither group knew which pill was being given.

The results: The placebo group's blood pressure stayed about the same without the drugs. In other words, although doctors had kept them on diuretics for years, they no longer appeared to need them.

Don't however, make any changes in your medication without medical guidance.

different people. "We would like to
be able to predict which drugs will
work," says Dr. Langford, "but for
now we have to operate according to
trial and error."

What this means is that your
doctor might have to prescribe several drugs or combinations of drugs
before he finds the one that is right
for you. So don't be alarmed if you
are switched from medication to
medication. "We like to think that a
person with not-too-severe hypertension will always be able to find a
drug that works, with minimal side
effects," says Dr. Langford.

The drugs are usually prescribed in a stepped sequence, after
diet therapy has been tried. Diuretics are given first, then a sympathetic inhibitor and then a vasodilator.
One in two people won't need more
than a diuretic. The remaining people will need multiple drugs. This
latter group shouldn't automatically
think that their illness is worse, just
that it is a little more complicated.
Remember, not everyone responds
the same way to the same drugs.

STICK TO TREATMENT PLAN

Once you and your doctor find the
right medication, take the drugs
according to schedule—*especially*
when you feel well. Many people
stop taking their drugs when they
feel good and trigger a possibly
dangerous relapse of high blood
pressure. If you forget to take your
medication for a couple of days,
don't try to make up for it by taking
the pills you missed. Instead, just
resume taking them according to the
schedule your doctor outlined. Once
back on the schedule, try to get into
a routine so you won't forget to take
your pills. Dr. Kaplan recommends
that if you take one a day, you
should take it in the morning, and
that if you take four a day, you
should take one before each meal
and at bedtime.

It's just as important to ask
your doctor to explain all the side
effects associated with your drug
therapy. Then if you feel bad, you'll
know when to contact your doctor.

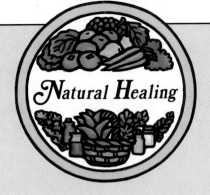

Natural Healing

In addition to drug therapy, there are many
natural ways to control high blood pressure without risking serious side effects. The following are
proven steps that should lead to lower blood
pressure. Of course, speak to your doctor before
making any changes in your pressure control
program. But chances are these natural treatments can be used right along with your drugs.

Take your blood pressure at home every day.
Studies show that you can track your treatment
better this way. Cut back on sodium, which may
be one of the most important contributors to high
blood pressure; watch for "hidden" salt in packaged and fast foods. Lose weight; you shed pressure as you shed pounds. Decaffeinate yourself or
at least cut back. Eat more onions and garlic, two
spices that can help lower blood pressure. Finally,
try to lead a calmer life. This may take some
practice, but you'll feel better for it. A dog or
cat might help. Studies show that pets help you
relax and give you a feeling of peace that will help
lower your blood pressure. In fact, even watching a
tank full of fish has been shown to help lower
blood pressure.

Side effects are a good sign that
your medication should be changed.
In any case, see your doctor periodically to make sure that your disease
hasn't become worse (maybe he'll tell
you you've improved!).

Meanwhile, try to make lifestyle
changes that help control blood pressure without drugs. Such changes
might make it possible for you to
stop or reduce your medication in
the future.

Infections

You're feeling pretty awful, so you go to your doctor. "Pneumonia," he says, casually tearing off a prescription for some weird-sounding drug. After a few weeks of taking the drug—and taking it easy—you feel great again. Serious, but it couldn't have been *that* serious, you think.

Wrong. Forty years ago, pneumonia could have killed you overnight. You've been saved by one of our most taken-for-granted heroes, an antibiotic. Antibiotics have conquered some of our meanest, deadliest enemies— leprosy, tuberculosis, scarlet fever, syphilis, to name a few — and infectious disease has dropped from *the* leading cause to the fifth leading cause of death in this country.

How important are they? Stuart Levy, M.D., professor of medicine, molecular biology and microbiology at Tufts University Medical School, says, "They have revolutionized medicine. They are the single agent that has most altered medical history."

Colonel Edmund Tramont, M.D., head of the U.S. Army's Infectious Disease Department, goes even further: "They are the cornerstone on which modern medicine is built."

Antibiotics are one part of a group of drugs called anti-infectives, which also include antifungals and antiviral drugs. Their names are self-explanatory. Antifungals can help clear up fungal infections, which range from serious lung diseases to itchy nuisances like athlete's foot. Antivirals, of course, battle viruses. But these cell-attackers aren't so easily dispatched—that's why you usually have to suffer through a cold or the flu—and so far, there's only one antiviral drug on the market (excluding herpes drugs).

Variety isn't lacking in antibiotics, though. Since their official discovery in 1928, many others have been found and used to knock out infections ranging from food poisoning to the once-fatal meningitis and Rocky Mountain spotted fever.

Penicillin and its derivatives (ampicillin, nafcillin, cloxacillin), the original antibiotics, are still the anti-infective of choice for most common bacterial infections because of their astonishing effectiveness, low cost and safety. Because allergic reactions are fairly common, however, many physicians use *tetracyclines* for a variety of infections, especially respiratory infections. If you take tetracyclines, completely avoid milk, cheese, ice cream and butter—these stymie the drug's effectiveness.

Aminoglycosides such as gentamycin and streptomycin are used for serious infections. Streptomycin, for example, is used to treat tuberculosis. These are strong medicines, and they can pack some pretty strong side effects. Severe nausea, vomiting and dizziness are not uncommon when taking streptomycin. In fact, people being treated with any aminoglycoside are kept under close medical observation because of potential toxicity. In other words, they are not popularly prescribed drugs.

Cephalosporins such as Keflex and Ceclor don't have any such popularity problems. Some 54 percent of all antibiotics prescribed are cephalosporins, and 10 million hospital patients took them last year. While most antibiotics have side effects or unwanted interactions with other drugs or foods, one of the biggest side effects of cephalosporins is on your wallet: They're expensive.

Macrolides such as erythromycin are used to treat children's ear, throat and skin infections, among other diseases. They were on their way to pharmacological oblivion in the 1970s when researchers noticed they were the only drugs that wouldn't take marching orders from Legionnaire's disease.

Other categories of antibiotics are *sulfa drugs,* which are used to treat urinary tract infections, and *polymyxins* and *chloramphenicol* which are used only for very serious infections.

If an infection is serious enough to land you in the hospital, brace yourself. A physican might have to inject you with an antibiotic, or use a combination of them.

"On an outpatient basis, however, an oral dose of a single antibiotic should be all that's required," says

Abusing a Miracle

With a global market of more than $1 billion, antibiotics make up the lion's share of the total profits for pharmaceutical companies. And prescriptions of antibiotics for the common cold abound despite the well-known fact that colds are viral diseases and thus cannot be touched by this class of drugs, which affects only bacterial disease.

Studies also show that in an astounding number of cases these drugs not only are misapplied, they also may be ineffective. A growing number of life-threatening diseases are now resistant to antibiotics, says Richard Novick, M.D., from New York City's Public Health Research Institute.

"There's no question that the widespread abuse of antibiotics at all levels of our society is leading to a backsliding in their effectiveness in treating disease," says Dr. Novick.

Why? Because antibiotics work by attacking and destroying *susceptible* strains of bacteria, any strain of bacteria that is not sensitive to antibiotics still remains alive. These resistant bacteria then multiply. Resistant bacteria can transfer the genetic information for their unique resistance to any other bacteria. Thus, antibiotics have scored initial wins against sensitive bacteria for many decades, but at the cost of leaving behind a clear field of resistant strains.

A generation ago, penicillin, for example, could be relied on to combat infections with up to 100 percent effectiveness. Today, drug companies market close to 300 varieties of penicillin, not only to fight a larger variety of bacteria but also to combat resistant forms of the same infections which only decades ago were seemingly under control.

And even these new varieties will become useless in the future. Calling for reductions in antibiotic use, physician and microbiologist Stuart Levy, M.D., warns that "microbes invulnerable to common medicine are gaining strength everywhere in the world because of the overuse of drugs such as tetracycline, ampicillin and chloramphenicol."

As the medical world wakens to the challenge of slowing the global antibiotic deluge, here are a few things you might do to prevent not only abuse but also infectious disease.

- If you must take antibiotics, be sure to observe timing and dosage instructions to the letter. This ensures the proper concentrations to kill the beasts; anything less leaves the job undone and will prolong your illness or endanger your life.
- Remember: Antibiotics are worthless against the common cold and other viruses.
- Don't share your prescription with friends or family.
- Avoid pressuring your doctor to hand out prescriptions. Ask for lab tests to be certain of the right antibiotic match for your illness. A wrong match can cause superinfections or kill harmless organisms, allowing resistant strains to overdevelop.

Being an informed consumer not only helps you personally but also helps to prevent the abuse of these truly effective drugs—helping them to have a use in the future.

Dr. Levy. "If you're prescribed more than one antibiotic, question it."

Remember, these drugs aren't candy, so use them judiciously. They're lifesavers that have rescued millions in the past half century. And they'll save millions more if we can keep the miracle in these miracle drugs by preventing their overuse.

Nervous System Diseases

A 19-year-old woman leans over to hug her boyfriend. Instead, she punches him in the back several times and passes out. She's not giving him mixed messages. Rather, her own brain messages are mixed, causing the involuntary thrashing movements called myoclonic jerks. She's one of two million Americans with epilepsy, a chronic nervous system disorder resulting from abnormal brain-wave patterns.

Epilepsy, cerebral palsy and Parkinson's disease are all disorders affecting different parts of the nervous system (which includes the brain, spinal cord and nerves). They are treated, to varying degrees, with drugs.

EPILEPSY

Epilepsy can result from anything that harms the brain—a brain injury before or at the time of birth, very high fevers during early childhood or infectious diseases such as mumps or measles. Seizures are the most common symptom and can range from mild twitches to violent convulsions that leave the victim unconscious.

Treatment may involve using anticonvulsant drugs. Doctors now are more and more likely to treat epilepsy with only one drug at a time, rather than using multiple drugs as they did in the past. Limiting medication to the single most effective drug seems to be the best way to control seizures with minimal side effects. First the doctor will determine which of the two basic seizure types the person is experiencing—either partial seizures involving a specific part of the brain or generalized seizures involving the whole brain.

Then he will select the correct medication, one intended to control a relatively specific seizure type.

SELECTION OF DRUGS

There are about eight commonly used drugs for treating epilepsy. Each works by a different mechanism, says one neurologist. For example,

he explains, "phenobarbital decreases the spread of a disturbance in the brain called an epileptogenic focus, which is what causes a seizure. Although the actual way that the drug Dilantin works has never been fully understood, it seems that it also decreases the possibility of this disturbance occurring in the brain, thus preventing a seizure."

If you take Dilantin, your doctor should periodically check your levels of folate, a B vitamin, because the drug may deplete this nutrient to the point where it *causes* seizures.

Some antiepileptic drugs may interact with each other. For example the drug carbamazepine (Tegretol) may decrease levels of both Dilantin and valproic acid. Conversely, phenobarbital and Dilantin may reduce blood levels of carbamazepine. A drug called Mysoline breaks down to phenobarbital and therefore should not be taken *with* phenobarbital because an average dose of the latter may then become toxic. Make sure your doctor—or your pharmacist, if you're seeing more than one physician—is aware of these interactions.

Some anticonvulsants also interact with such common substances as antacids, vitamin D and cimetidine, an ulcer drug. Phenobarbital, Dilantin and carbamazepine can decrease the effectiveness of oral contraceptives and the blood thinner warfarin. Again, check with your doctor or pharmacist for the possibility of interactions.

CEREBRAL PALSY

Cerebral palsy, a partial paralysis caused by damaged nerve tissue, affects about 700,000 people in the United States. It is a neuromuscular disorder caused by brain damage that occurs before, at the time of or immediately after birth. Poor development or severe damage to one half of the brain results in very weak or almost totally paralyzed muscles on the opposite side of the body.

The primary treatment for cerebral palsy is not usually drugs, but rather physical therapy or rehabilitation. Sometimes brain surgery may prove beneficial. Medication, however, is used to try to reduce spasticity. "By and large, they're not terribly effective medications," says a neurologist at Washington University School of Medicine, St. Louis. "They work by a variety of mechanisms, but they're not satisfactory because they often produce side effects and do not produce a lot of benefits."

"Dantrium has a lot of side effects," says a neurologist, "the most dangerous being liver toxicity. Baclofen is a much safer drug."

PARKINSON'S DISEASE

Parkinson's disease first affects its victims usually around the age of 50 or 60, although it may appear as early as 30. In his book, *Your Brain and Nerves,* J. Lawrence Pool, M.D., reports on a patient who came to him with early symptoms of the disease. The man "almost got into a fight because a man at an adjacent restaurant table accused him of winking at his girl," writes Dr. Pool. The uncontrollably blinking eyelid was a form of spasmodic muscle contraction, a characteristic of Parkinson's disease.

More common symptoms of Parkinson's disease include progressive stiffness of the muscles, making walking difficult; stiffness of facial muscles, creating a "deadpan" appearance known as a masked face; and a rhythmic to-and-fro tremor of the arms. Drugs are one of the main therapies for Parkinson's disease. They reduce rigidity and make it easier for the person to move.

"Every person responds differently to the medication," says one neurologist. "The drug that consistently works the best is Sinemet, which took the place of the old levodopa, which had a common side effect of nausea and vomiting because of the large doses necessary to get even a small amount into the brain."

Sinemet combines carbidopa with levodopa and allows the patient to take much less levodopa, since the former forces more of the latter into the brain. Some side effects

of levodopa are a change in blood pressure (usually lowered) and abnormal movements.

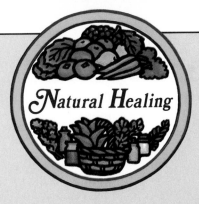

Natural Healing

If you have any one of the nervous system disorders discussed here, the following might help you find your own means of natural control:

- Medical research indicates that choline (a nutrient in the B complex group) may work to reduce convulsions.
- Vitamins B_6, and E and the minerals manganese, magnesium and calcium also have been shown to help prevent epileptic seizures or reduce their frequency.
- The frequency of seizures also can be lessened by getting a good night's sleep, says James F. Toole, M.D., professor of neurology, Bowman Gray School of Medicine, North Carolina. To achieve blissful slumber he suggests getting enough exercise to produce physical fatigue.
- Dr. Toole also advises little or no alcohol consumption for epileptic persons, as it makes seizures more likely to occur. Alcohol also exaggerates the side effects of the barbiturates and anticonvulsant drugs taken for epilepsy.
- If you suffer from Parkinson's disease, try keeping limber by moving stiff muscles and joints. Bending, stretching and walking are all good activities, says Dr. Toole. If you are taking levodopa, he recommends avoiding a high-protein diet because it may interfere with this drug.
- Those with cerebral palsy were less spastic and seemed to function better and feel better in general when one doctor put them on a regimen of supplements of vitamins and minerals to counter any deficiencies discovered during examination. (People with nervous system disorders should use nutritional supplements only under the supervision of a doctor.)

Pain

When illness or injury strikes, it's usually pain that makes us rush for aid. Should a child wake in the middle of the night suffering from nausea, the parents are likely to sit out the illness until morning. But if the same child wakes with a painful ear infection, the parents are likely to rush the screaming child to the hospital.

Pain is an insistent warning that something is wrong. Most pain can be directly traced to a tissue or nerve injury. And while it's vital to know when and where we have been injured, once the message has been delivered, we'd like the messenger to leave.

When cells are injured—say you hit your thumb with a hammer while building a dog house or pull a muscle while riding your bike—the cells signal your brain by releasing chemicals that tell your nerve endings to pay attention. These nerves in turn alert the brain that some-thing is wrong. It's much the same as someone who sees smoke sending a signal from a firebox on the street to a fire station. When the signal reaches the brain, you feel pain.

You can attempt to control this pain in two basic ways: by keeping the injured cells from signaling your brain or by masking the way your brain responds to the signal. While it might be best never to feel pain, it is sometimes too difficult to stop the pain at its source. So you resort to something that disguises or masks it.

We most frequently find this type of relief from pain in drugs, but meditation, massage, electrical stimulation and hypnosis also work. The reason drugs are sometimes the therapy of choice is because they work quickly and conveniently and are (in the short run, at least) safe. These pain drugs are called analgesics and come in two basic types: narcotic analgesics like morphine, and nonnarcotic analgesics like aspirin, acetaminophen and ibuprofen.

The narcotic analgesics tend to work in a big, sometimes numbing way to relieve you of pain. They work on the whole central nervous system to make your pain less distressing. (Nonnarcotic drugs generally work to stop your nerves from transmitting pain messages in the first place.) Still, while the narcotic drugs, including Percodan, codeine, morphine and Demerol, are effective, they are also linked to some very serious side effects.

Nelson Hendler, M.D., assistant professor of neurosurgery at John Hopkins University School of Medicine, who runs the Mensano Pain Clinic in Stevenson, Maryland, says that "narcotics can be very useful for severe pain following surgery and for short-term pain, but they pose problems in the long run." At his clinic he deals mostly with people who suffer chronic pain, and he never prescribes narcotics. He considers the long-term side effects undesirable. These include the sexual problems, gastrointestinal difficulties and impaired thinking that sometimes occur in patients who take the drugs for more than a month or so.

Results Are Better When Patients Control Their Own Painkillers

Let postsurgery patients control their own painkillers? No way, right? They're apt to drug themselves into oblivion.

Well, that belief—that patients in pain need doctors to dole out just the right amount of relief—was debunked by doctors at the University of Kentucky College of Medicine, who gave one group of patients the responsibility of administering their own medication during a 60-hour period following surgery. Meanwhile, another group of patients was given medication in the normal way, every 4 to 6 hours as needed. The results: 92 percent of the self-medicators reported satisfactory pain relief, compared to only 58 percent of the traditional group.

You might assume the reason the do-it-yourself group fared so well is that they took plenty of drugs to kill the pain. They actually used *less* medication than the doctor-controlled group.

With narcotics, there is also the possibility that a patient will become addicted if the drugs are administered for a long period of time, say a month or longer. After all, prescribed narcotics have the same chemical base as heroin. If a person becomes addicted to a prescribed narcotic, the doctor can provide medical supervision to break the addiction, but withdrawal is not pleasant and the whole problem is best avoided. Many physicians have their patients take other drugs or use alternatives to drug therapy if they are suffering from chronic pain that requires long-term treatment.

Two fairly recent narcoticlike drugs that are gaining in favor are Stadol and Nuban, which are called agonist/antagonists. "That's confusing, of course," says Dr. Hendler, "but basically what it means is that the drugs stimulate the narcotic receptors, but not too much, so you don't have a full-blown narcotic effect."

Still, these drugs can cause problems. They are similar in action to Talwin, a drug that has been around for quite a while. It is widely used even though it is associated with some problems. If it is repeatedly injected, it will damage the skin. "This can be prevented, obviously, by not using the drug by injection," says Dr. Hendler. Another side effect, hallucinations, can't be predicted, but doctors feel it is a rare occurrence, so Talwin is commonly prescribed.

Stadol and Nuban also are parenteral drugs, meaning they must be taken by injection, but they don't cause the same skin damage as Talwin. Still, although they aren't classified as addictive, Dr. Hendler says his experience with patients shows that they can be habit forming.

A commonly prescribed analgesic drug which *is* classified as a narcotic, and acts on the same receptors as morphine, is Darvon. While many doctors use this drug—which comes in three forms—for patients suffering from mild to moderately severe pain, Dr. Hendler says that the relief may be due more to the dose of aspirin found in the Darvon compounds (Darvon Compound or Darvon with A.S.A.) than to the prescrip-

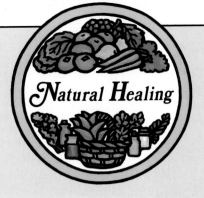

Natural Healing

People with pain, especially if it is long-term pain, often don't want to rely on drug therapy. Fortunately, there are several effective nondrug pain relievers. One is transcutaneous electrical nerve stimulation, a daunting name for an effective pain reliever known by the acronym TENS. With TENS, the patient actually gives the area that hurts mild jolts of electricity which, in effect, distract the nervous system from feeling severe pain. The electricity also causes the brain to produce above-normal amounts of endorphins and other natural painkillers produced by the body. While TENS isn't a cure-all, it might be worth your while to ask about this treatment.

Other natural techniques include massage; heat to relieve muscle pain; cold to numb incidental pain; or acupuncture or acupressure. Of course, check with your doctor before trying any new pain-relief methods to see if they're safe for your condition.

Finally, gentle exercise such as stretching is a time-tested way to help relieve minor pains. And regular exercise is a great way to prevent pain in the future.

tion chemical, propoxyphene, that is supposed to make Darvon unique. Darvon, like the other pain drugs, is associated with so many side effects that you should have a serious discussion with your doctor about whether or not you really need it.

In fact, because there are so many possible side effects from various painkillers, you should always discuss a range of options with your doctor.

Skin Diseases

Sometimes the disease that's hardest to take is the one that shows itself off to everyone around you. That's what makes diseases of the skin, like chronic acne, eczema and that old heartbreak, psoriasis, so miserable for people who have them. But luckily—even with a life-long condition like psoriasis—correct use of the right drugs can provide relief that's at least skin deep.

Frederick Urbach, M.D., is professor and chairman of dermatology as well as director of the Skin and Cancer Center at Philadelphia's Temple University. He explains that dermatologists not only use medications that are applied directly to the skin but often prescribe drugs taken internally.

ANTIBIOTIC ATTACK

Antibiotics, for example, are used to combat bacterial infections of the skin like impetigo. But Dr. Urbach points out that they are more frequently used to treat secondary infections such as those that develop when bacteria get into the broken skin of the eczema sufferer to compound the problem with an infection.

"The bacteria didn't cause the disease," he explains, "but you're not going to get the underlying problem better until you get the infection cleared up."

And there's a third use for these drugs in cases (like acne) where bacteria aren't the cause and there isn't an infection, but where bacteria aggravate the disease.

And, Dr. Urbach says, there are even situations where antibiotics have an effect that is *not* due to any killing of bacteria. An example is seborrheic dermatitis, an extremely common skin disorder of the scalp and face that seems to respond very well to an antibiotic used to treat yeast infections. "Nobody's sure why it works," admits Dr. Urbach, "but there are situations where one uses internal drugs based on the experience that they help without knowing exactly how they do it."

PUTTING OUT THE FIRE

The second most widely used oral medications in skin care are corticosteroids like prednisone and triamcinolone. These are used to calm an inflammation. "If you have a disease

---

Accutane: Not for Pregnant Women

Accutane has become practically synonymous with birth defects, and it's one of the very few drugs to be labeled with the FDA's strongest possible warning under the new safety-during-pregnancy code (see "Are Your Drugs Rated X?" on page 94).

The problem with this acne medication is that it's generally prescribed for young people who are at their peak of sexual activity. When pregnancy and Accutane collide, everyone agrees that birth defects can be the result. The manufacturer's warnings to physicians include instructions that contraception *must* be used by female patients, but Frederick Urbach, M.D., of Temple University, explains that, luckily, the disease is much more common in the male of the species. "We don't use it for women unless it's the *only* thing we can use. There are usually some alternatives we can try. They're not as good, but Accutane use in women can be a real hazard."

The company's own literature warns that almost everyone who uses the drug will experience dry skin, especially dry and cracked lips, during the 4-month course of treatment. In addition, there is a laundry list of possible side effects, including disturbing reports about possible skeletal changes that include bony growths in long-term users.

But, as Dr. Urbach points out, "severe cystic acne is an extremely deforming disease that can go on for years and leave permanent scars. Nobody dies from acne, so Accutane isn't a lifesaving drug, but it's a mind saver that spares the sufferer the scars and mental stress."

that's highly inflamed, these are the drugs that help treat it," explains Dr. Urbach. He uses the example of an unfortunate soul with a horrible case of poison ivy. "You either give him prednisone for two weeks or send him to the hospital for ten days." Dr. Urbach cautions, however, that milder drugs are preferable when the disease isn't "really terrible."

Dr. Urbach explains that using oral corticosteroids would be an "unusual" treatment for diseases that are not inflammatory, such as acne.

To give these drugs for a long time in a "lifetime disease" like psoriasis could cause serious side effects, he says.

When corticosteroids are used topically on the skin, Dr. Urbach finds "by and large no chronic side effects, except with very long use in some areas, where they may cause thinning of the skin—and that only occurs after many years." He feels that these topical preparations are quite safe when used wisely and are effective in treating various forms of eczema, contact dermatitis and "the hand rashes people get when their hands are always in water."

Generally, a thin film of ointment will do the job. In certain circumstances, where extra penetration is desired, the affected area will be covered with Saran Wrap (or any waterproof food wrap). But because of the extra absorption, Dr. Urbach warns that this should be done only under the control of a physician.

Despite the safety of topical preparations, Dr. Urbach cautions, "A doctor should check the patient every six months to a year to make sure the drug is still working effectively." He explains that patients can develop a resistance to one of the many formulas available and require a change, or may improve to the point where the dosage can be reduced.

Another drug effective in treating psoriasis is coal tar. It's not used as extensively as it once was, mostly because "people don't accept that black, sticky stuff on the skin anymore." This drug, too, Dr. Urbach warns, must be used with supervision, because of possible side effects

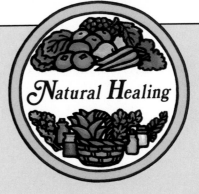

Natural Healing

A report from Sweden suggests that oral zinc supplements may be just as effective as tetracycline in clearing up complexions marred by acne. The zinc treatment averaged an impressive 70 percent improvement after 12 weeks. In another study, the effects of zinc were compared to those of vitamin A, from which the drug Accutane is derived. A dose of 135 milligrams of zinc was significantly more effective at clearing up faces than amounts of vitamin A so massive they would be extremely dangerous. As with many treatments, no one is really sure why it works, but some feel that acne is related to a deficiency in zinc. (Take large amounts of zinc only under a doctor's supervision.)

like irritation and inflammation of hair follicles.

NEW ACNE TREATMENTS

The controversial acne medication Accutane (see "Accutane: Not for Pregnant Women") is considered safe when used correctly, but, Dr. Urbach says, it should be reserved only for very severe cases in which the patient is literally deformed by the disease and the treatment is supervised by a dermatologist. "There are other ways to treat milder acne; benzoyl peroxide, for instance, can be very effective," he explains.

One type of drug that isn't often prescribed for skin problems is tranquilizers. Dr. Urbach believes that more emotional problems are caused by skin disorders than the other way around. "Not only that, tranquilizers should be prescribed by someone who knows how to use them. A dermatologist shouldn't try to be a psychiatrist," he says.

9

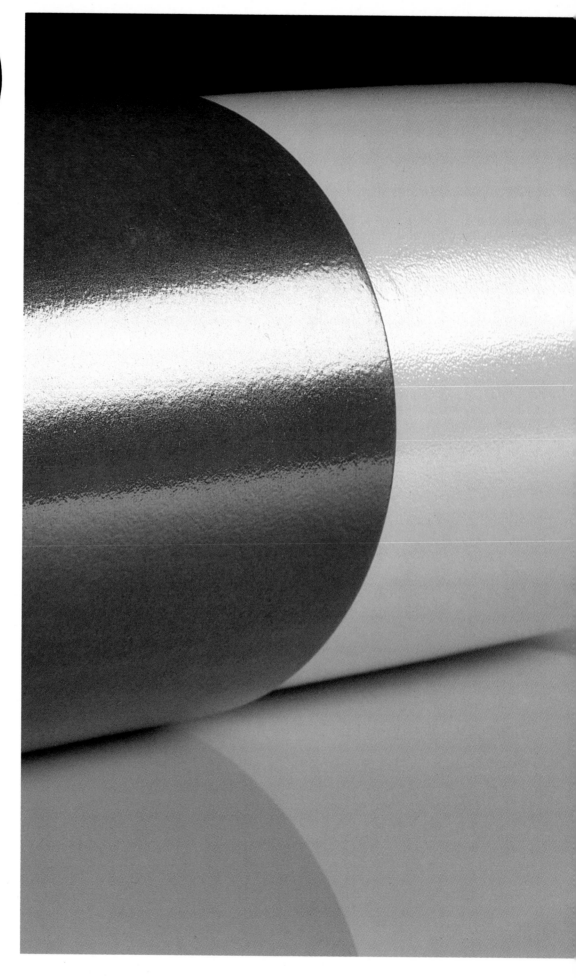

The Power of the Placebo

The most potent medicine of all is found right in your own mind.

Faster than a speeding microbe! More powerful than a local morphine! Able to leap tall infections in a single bound! Is it a bird? Is it a plane? No, it's—Superpill!

You're skeptical? You think superheroes belong only on Saturday morning cartoons and superdrugs only in historical reports about old-time cures with names like "My Amazing Gray-Colored Tonic" (guaranteed to cure any ache and strip old paint from furniture, depending on which you might have more need for)? Well, suppose we told you that there *is* a Wonder Drug. It's available everywhere. It's inexpensive. And it's *immensely* powerful. In fact, this intrepid drug can single-handedly combat your high blood pressure, your low pain tolerance, your headaches, insomnia, allergies, sniffles, psychoses and any severe case of the "blues." It can make you fatter; it can make you thinner. It can heal you almost instantly, or it can inhibit healing altogether. Its unique power enables Tibetan Buddhists to raise their body temperature enough so that snow melts into little puddles around them. Its unique virulence produced toxic symptoms in Tylenol users *nationwide* after poisoned Tylenol was found—only—in Chicago. It is the most powerful drug known to man, and the least understood. It can cure almost any illness; but there is almost no illness it can't also cause. What is it, this amazing Superdrug? Why, it is the potent, the mysterious, the fearsome . . . sugar pill.

Yes, the sugar pill. Or, in more general terms—the potent, mysterious and fearsome placebo *(plah-SEE-bow)*. Medicine's most multitalented cure-all, the placebo can actually take any form. Many of us imagine (and dismiss) it as just some sugar-coated, comforting, useless pill. But a placebo is, technically, any kind of treatment that shouldn't have a specific effect on the illness being treated but that, somehow, does.

WHY "WORTHLESS" TREATMENT CAN WORK

Any substance or treatment can have a strong placebo effect. The simple act of giving an injection, for example, can be an effective placebo. In Nigeria a special breed of "doctor" travels about, injecting his patients with waters colored red, yellow or blue (different colors at different prices). He charges a lot of money, and lines of willing patients form wherever he goes. The result? In an especially colorful example of the placebo effect in action, many of these patients get complete relief from their water shot. "The fact is that you could prescribe bottled dish water to be used as an eyewash once daily and achieve a 30 to 50 percent improvement" in people with cataracts, one doctor has, rather ruefully, admitted.

He shouldn't be surprised. The placebo effect has existed for as long as healing has. And healing has existed for as long as humanity has (otherwise we would have succumbed early on to the dangers of damp caves and feisty predators). Early healing, though, had little to do with "medicine." It had nothing to do with science. Witch doctors, bizarre rituals and remedies that ranged from the quaint to the nauseating (see "Take Two Frog Eyes and Call Me in the Morning") were all that

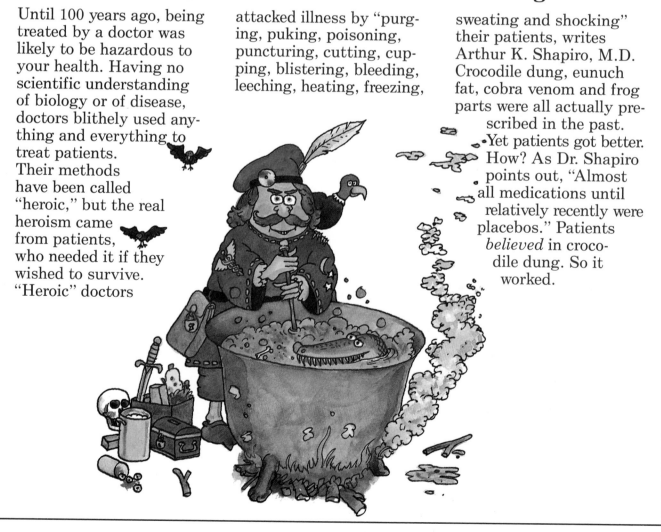

"Take Two Frog Eyes and Call Me in the Morning . . . "

Until 100 years ago, being treated by a doctor was likely to be hazardous to your health. Having no scientific understanding of biology or of disease, doctors blithely used anything and everything to treat patients. Their methods have been called "heroic," but the real heroism came from patients, who needed it if they wished to survive. "Heroic" doctors attacked illness by "purging, puking, poisoning, puncturing, cutting, cupping, blistering, bleeding, leeching, heating, freezing, sweating and shocking" their patients, writes Arthur K. Shapiro, M.D. Crocodile dung, eunuch fat, cobra venom and frog parts were all actually prescribed in the past. Yet patients got better. How? As Dr. Shapiro points out, "Almost all medications until relatively recently were placebos." Patients *believed* in crocodile dung. So it worked.

our forefathers had to treat their illnesses and injuries. Their healing practices shared only one important aspect: They shouldn't have worked. But often they did. They worked only because the patients' *belief* in them made them work. They worked only because they were placebos. "From antiquity to this era of medical enlightenment, [the] placebo has been the single most potent and versatile tool for relieving the sufferings man is heir to," a report published in the *Mayo Clinic Proceedings* concluded. "Be it mother's kiss or voodoo drums, leeches, purgatives, poultices or snake oil, the wondrous effect of placebo therapy is undeniably evident." Or, as Arthur K. Shapiro, M.D., of Mt. Sinai Hospital in New York, a pioneer placebo researcher, has more bluntly said, "The history of medical treatment. . .[is] the history of the placebo effect."

Medicine and medical men have not always been eager to acknowledge this. The word *placebo* (from the Latin verb meaning "to please") didn't even appear in a medical textbook until 1811, when it was defined as "any medicine adapted more to please than benefit the patient." Its reputation has been degenerating ever since. Until very recently, in fact, the placebo effect tended to be dismissed as incidental, imaginary, unfortunate or what happens when you give dummy pills to dummies.

DUMMY PILLS AND THE DOUBLE-BLIND

The only function that "scientific" medicine had been willing to give to the placebo was as the "useless thing" against which "real medicine" is measured in double-blind testing. First used by the FDA in 1962 to test the effectiveness of prescription drugs, double-blind testing is a procedure in which patients are given either a drug or a placebo. They don't know which they're getting. Neither does their doctor. The patients' reactions are then measured.

If it's decided that the drug is "no more effective than a placebo," it's all over for that drug: It's pulled

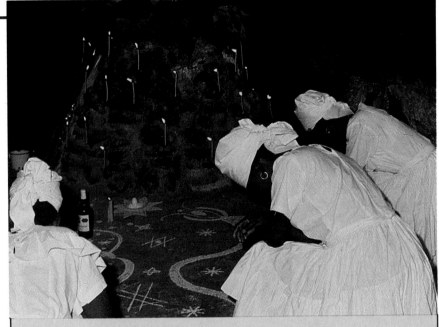

Voodoo—A Fatal Faith

Dolls strategically stabbed. Pounding drums. Weird chants. Smoke. Moaning. Bones. The stuff of which B movies are made? Maybe. But also the lethal props of witch doctors who literally do "scare their victims to death." In a famed 1957 report on voodoo, Walter Cannon, M.D., formerly a Harvard physiologist, found that "the belief that one has been subjected to sorcery. . .does actually result in death in the course of time."

Among other documented stories, he tells of robust Australian warriors who had a bone pointed at them threateningly and later died. Nothing was physically wrong with them: They died of self-induced shock. The fear—and faith—in the mind of a cursed victim can be so strong, they become deadly.

from the market. Hundreds of drugs were abolished after double-blind testing was first introduced. Most of these drugs had, seemingly, been working fine until then. Many of them had produced cures. But how could that be if they were "ineffective"? Few people in the medical community, it seems, had given much thought to *why* placebos work.

Unfortunately, even today most doctors simply don't know very much at all about the placebo. The subject is almost completely ignored in medical schools. Of 19 popular textbooks currently used in medical schools,

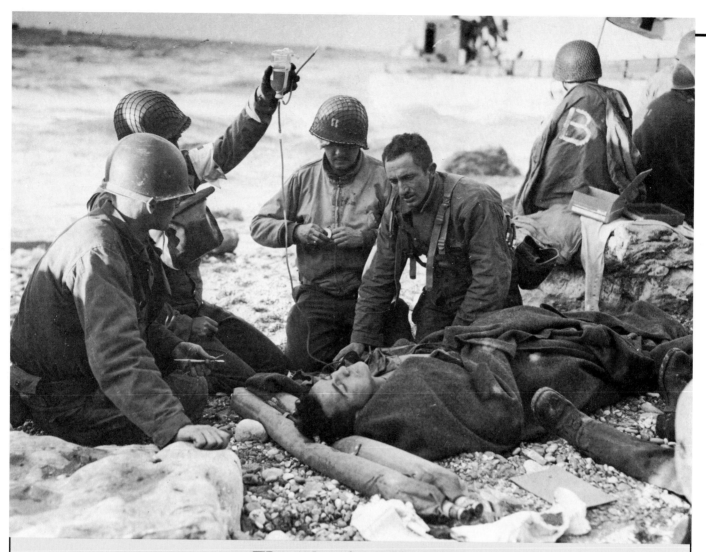

The "Anzio Effect"

You know the scene: A sweet-faced young soldier smiles heroically, claiming that his dreadful wound "doesn't hurt at all," while nurses coo sympathetically and John Wayne pats him on the shoulder. Perhaps you dismissed it as one more silly Hollywood invention. But during World War II, Henry Beecher, M.D., formerly of Harvard Medical School, made a discovery that makes those sappy Hollywood scenes seem like a documentary: Only a quarter of the seriously wounded soldiers in a specific combat zone, including those on the beachhead at Anzio, Italy, asked for pain relief. The others claimed not to need any. Yet their wounds were as severe as or more severe than those suffered by postoperative patients whom Dr. Beecher attended after the war.

Three-fourths of these patients clamored for morphine.

What kept the soldiers pain free? Dr. Beecher decided that the so-called Anzio effect was the result of a soldier's *expectations*. For him a serious wound was a wonderful thing, a free ticket back "to the safety of the hospital." According to Dr. Beecher, his wound released him from "an exceedingly dangerous environment." So he became "euphoric."

What all of this means is that pain is a function of the body *and* mind. And it was this fact that led Dr. Beecher to the scientific discovery of the placebo: When people *believed* a pill would relieve their pain, it often did—even if it was made of sugar. The "Anzio effect" had become the "placebo effect."

only 3 even mention the placebo, and each of these only in passing. Studies have also shown that three-fourths of all doctors still think the placebo effect is something that happens in *other* doctors' practices, not in their own. The very word, for them, smacks of unsavory hocus-pocus, of quackery. "The placebo effect is a neglected and berated asset of patient care," Herbert Benson, M.D., of Harvard Medical School, says.

As a result, the placebo effect also may at times be misused and abused. A survey of doctors and nurses recently completed by researchers at the University of New Mexico School of Medicine found that the majority of them badly underestimated the power of the placebo. Most believed its effect to be imaginary, a proof that the patient's problem wasn't "real." They tended, therefore to use placebos as a kind of punishment, giving them to patients who were disruptive or unpopular. If the patient responded to the placebo, the staff took this as evidence of psychiatric problems. If he didn't respond. . . .well, maybe they hadn't liked him to begin with, so who cared?

SUGAR PILLS CAN HELP PATIENTS

All of which is not merely callous, but is approaching the tragic, because it means that many of us are being denied a potential "wonder drug." And wonderful it is; as more and more scientific research is done, less and less doubt remains that placebos are among the most powerful of all medications. "There is no direct physical response of the human body to any therapeutic procedure that cannot occur with equal form and magnitude in response to an inert placebo," Andrew Weil, M.D., an instructor at the University of Arizona College of Medicine, wrote in his book *Health and Healing*. Dr. Shapiro agrees. "Psychological or placebo effects can be. . .excluded if the dosage of a drug is high enough to cause. . .death," he says. But at any less drastic level, placebo effects play a big role. Studies have shown

Can Surgery Be a Placebo?

Surgery as a placebo? It hardly seems possible that something so certifiably "medical," so seemingly free from the influence of the patient's mind, could be a placebo. But medical history says it's so. Here's the story.

In the 1950s, surgical treatment for angina pectoris (intense chest pain that usually indicates a heart problem) became fashionable. The surgery involved opening the sufferer's chest and tying off the arteries that supply blood to the chest area. This was major surgery. It was traumatic. And it was successful: Up to 75 percent of patients reported lessened pain.

But in the late 1950s a few skeptical surgeons got sneaky and decided to test the effectiveness of the operations (in a way that would not be considered ethical today). They divided patients into two groups and told them they were going to undergo "wonder surgery." One group actually had the operation. The other group was anesthetized, had their chests opened and. . .that's all. Later, both groups were told they'd been successfully treated. *But the group who had had only a sham operation showed as much relief of symptoms as the group who'd been operated on.* Conclusion? The "real" surgery was, in fact, a placebo! The patients themselves created their recovery. Of course, those who'd had the full, major surgery had a lot more to recover from.

Not surprisingly, embarrassed surgeons quickly and quietly stopped doing surgery for angina. But some doctors now question whether they haven't replaced it with yet another surgical placebo: the coronary bypass.

that up to three-fourths of all patients who see their doctors will get better if they are given a placebo and only a placebo. "Even in the other 25 percent," Dr. Benson believes, "medical treatments may be enhanced by the placebo effect."

The immense power of the "dummy pill" wasn't clearly substantiated, though, until the mid-1950s. In a famous review of placebo studies, Henry Beecher, M.D., formerly of Harvard Medical School, reported that placebos can be effective more than 35 percent of the time in patients suffering from complaints as diverse as wound pain, seasickness, headaches and the common cold.

Even more amazing was Dr. Beecher's discovery that a plain old placebo can relieve pain almost as well as morphine can. In Dr. Beecher's study, patients who had just undergone surgery were divided into two groups, each receiving two doses of morphine alternating with two placebos. The first group received morphine, followed later by a placebo. The second group received the placebo first. Not surprisingly, the morphine was effective with the first dose, relieving pain in 52 percent of the patients. But the placebo was virtually as effective; 40 percent of the patients reported pain relief after receiving the first dose. The placebo's effectiveness, therefore, was 77 percent that of morphine—and this against pain that was undoubtedly real.

Doctors have admitted to being "dumbfounded" by these studies.

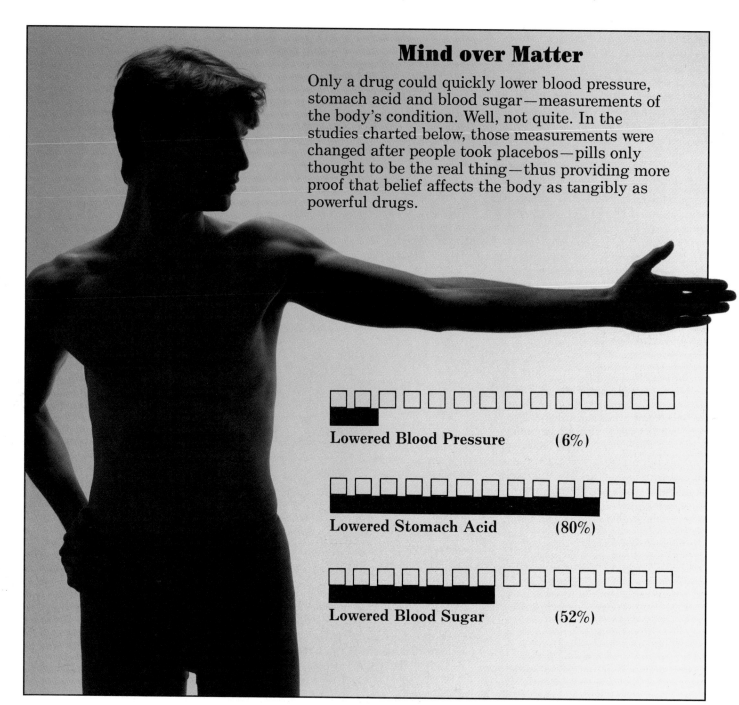

Mind over Matter

Only a drug could quickly lower blood pressure, stomach acid and blood sugar—measurements of the body's condition. Well, not quite. In the studies charted below, those measurements were changed after people took placebos—pills only thought to be the real thing—thus providing more proof that belief affects the body as tangibly as powerful drugs.

Lowered Blood Pressure (6%)

Lowered Stomach Acid (80%)

Lowered Blood Sugar (52%)

But, thousands of reports since have substantiated the power of the placebo. Considering that the word *placebo* didn't make its first appearance in a medical journal article until 1945, the sheer volume of research now available is a little breathtaking. Luckily, placebos themselves are breath-giving; sugar pills can, literally, clear your lungs. In other words, asthma responds to placebo treatment, as does that bane of most medical treatments, the common cold. Placebos also have been proven to relieve anxiety, motion sickness, premenstrual syndrome, chronic headaches, migraines, peptic ulcer pain and the nausea that may accompany radiation therapy. Placebos have helped insomniacs to sleep and depressed patients to revive.

PLACEBOS CAN AFFECT EVERY PART OF YOU

"Placebo effects are not imaginary, and may involve almost any organ," an article in the *Canadian Medical Association Journal* asserts. After being given a placebo, people have shown demonstrable changes in their stomach acidity, their blood pressure, their pupil size, their white blood cell levels and, among diabetics, in their blood sugar levels. Most of these effects, doctors had thought, were dependent on the use of strong drugs. But we now know that a placebo can mimic the effect of any drug.

In one especially interesting experiment to determine the effectiveness of double-blind studies, medical students—who, of all people, would probably consider themselves least susceptible to "unscientific hocus-pocus"—were given either nitroglycerine, a potent drug, or a placebo. Some students had no idea what they were receiving. Other students were told whether their dose was nitroglycerine or a placebo. *Both* substances decreased the students' blood pressure and caused their heartbeat to race.

The changes were greater among the students who were told they received the active drug; being medical students, they knew what to expect from it. However, those under the double-blind technique got the same degree of response from the placebo as from the nitroglycerine. Thinking they *may* have received the nitroglycerine, they *expected* their blood pressure to drop and their heart to flutter.

Expectations about drugs' effects can work just as dramatically in reverse. In an experiment again using medical students as subjects, the students were made to feel temporary, mild pain. Then they were given injections of meperidine, a strong narcotic. All of them received a good, stiff dose of the drug. It should have kept them blissfully pain free for some time. But at the same time that they received the injections, the students were told that some of the doses were placebos. What was their reaction? Well, when tests were done to measure their pain tolerance, in two-thirds of the cases the supposedly potent drug either had no effect at all or it *lowered* the students' pain tolerance. Pharmacology textbooks would swear up and down that meperidine should have done the opposite.

HOW BELIEF STRUCTURES HEALING

An even more startling example of the power of our beliefs occurred some years ago in a study by Stewart Wolf, M.D. Dr. Wolf, then affiliated with New York Hospital, treated a woman in the early stages of pregnancy. She was complaining of nausea and vomiting. Dr. Wolf sympathized with the woman and finally ordered the mother-to-be some medicine. He assured her that it would quickly clear up her nausea. Sure enough, it did. Within 20 minutes, her discomfort disappeared and did not reoccur until the following morning.

Dr. Wolf's mighty—and certainly controversial—remedy was ipecac, one of the strongest emetics known to man (or mother). It is usually given in cases of poisoning, in order to *cause* vomiting. But, in this case, it made the woman's sickness go away. How?

"People's expectations of drugs often explain their responses to them better than books of pharmacology," says Dr. Weil. "Belief is the key to these mysteries; not intellectual convictions but gut-level belief that links up with the physical nervous system and, through it, influences all the functions of the body."

Suppose you are prone to asthma, for example. Suddenly, one day you find yourself choking. You *cannot* breathe. You gasp, desperate for air. Luckily, you've had the good sense to do all this in the presence of a quick-thinking physician, one who is well versed in psychology. She steps up and shoots a needleful of salt water into your arm. She is calm, efficient and compassionate, assuring you that things will be fine. Your terror immediately eases, and your lungs open. Was it the salt water that did it? Hardly. It was *you*. *You* set in motion the chemical reactions that allowed your lungs to function easily again. The salt water didn't hurt. But it couldn't directly help, either.

Perhaps the name placebo effect itself needs to be changed. As it is, it implies that the placebo creates the cure; actually, *you* do. Jerome D. Frank, M.D., Ph.D., a professor emeritus of psychiatry at Johns Hopkins University School of Medicine, suggests that the "unfortunate term 'placebo effect'" is more like the "healing power of expectant faith."

Of course, the "healing power of expectant faith" doesn't have quite the snap and zing of the "placebo effect." But it does have the virtue of accuracy. "Negative emotions. . . can impede healing and positive ones such as expectant faith can enhance it," Dr. Frank writes in the *Johns Hopkins Medical Journal*. In an interesting study of patients about to undergo surgery on their detached retinas, it was found that those who scored high on an "acceptance test" —those who had faith in their surgeons and who expected the operation to be successful—recovered faster than the less optimistic patients.

Of course, the "healing power of expectant faith" has always had its most dramatic illustration at miracle shrines, the sites of so many "miraculous" cures. There, crippled people throw away their crutches and walk unaided. People with severe arthritis recover their flexibility and lose their pain. Medical science may dismiss these cures as either hoaxes or freak occurrences. But at the shrine in Lourdes, France, the "miracles" have been well documented. "The evidence that an occasional cure of advanced organic disease *does* occur at Lourdes is as strong as that for any other phenomenon accepted as true," Dr. Frank says.

But you don't have to go to Lourdes to find this kind of miraculous healing. In a study of cancer patients nationwide, 176 of them showed spontaneous remission of their disease, though they were receiving no treatment of any kind.

AMAZIN' GRACE

Faith, as in "faith healing," was also given an interesting test in a case reported by Dr. Frank in his book *Persuasion and Healing*. In this instance, a well-known local faith healer was asked by a physician to try to cure three of his patients from a distance, without their knowledge. The patients were all women and all were severely ill. One had chronic gallbladder inflammation with stones; the second, described as "practically a skeleton," had not as yet recovered from major abdominal surgery; the third was dying of cancer.

Well, the faith healer did his thing from afar. Nothing happened. The doctor then told his patients about the faith healer, leading them to believe that this particular healer was capable of miraculous cures. The doctor named a particular time and said the healer would be hard at work then. At the correct time all three women "improved dramatically." The woman who had undergone abdominal surgery was permanently cured. The cancer patient recovered enough that she could return home to her housework. The gallbladder patient also lost her symptoms and was soon able to go home. All were convinced that the healer had helped them. But—the healer was not working at the time they thought he was! The only logical conclusion is that, as Dr. Weil says, "one person cannot heal another any more than a muddy lake or an icy stream can." It is only

Placebos: A Double-Edged Sword

Anything packed into a pill can pack a powerful wallop, if you believe it can. That's why placebos are so potent and why even those made of "harmless" substances can produce all the toxic side effects of any potent pill. People on placebos have become sick, dizzy, itchy, faint, headachy, nauseated and plagued with intestinal disorders, among other symptoms. In more than one case, a person has become completely addicted to the "drug," requiring ever greater dosages and going through withdrawal when the placebo therapy was stopped.

Color Me Cured

Can the color of a drug—a nonmedicinal dye no more powerful than candy coating—make it work better? Yes, say scientists from two Alabama universities. They came to that conclusion after showing students medications of various colors and asking them to identify each. Yellow, orange or black capsules were expected to be stimulants. Light blue capsules were pegged as weak sedatives. And, probably because of aspirin advertising, white capsules were seen as painkillers. (Students were most in agreement about lavender capsules. Anything that color, they decided, must be a hallucinogen.)

a person's belief in outside practitioners or miracle shrines that gives them any power over illness."

YOUR HEALING POWER CAN ALSO HURT

"Happy" miracles don't always happen, though. The power that your faith and belief can generate is immense, but it is also neutral; it doesn't necessarily heal you. It can as easily harm you, depending on how you direct it. Dennis T. Jaffe, Ph.D., a psychologist affiliated with the Saybrook Institute Center for Health Studies in San Francisco, tells of just such a case in his book *Healing from Within*. A man suffering from terminal cancer heard about the wonderful healing properties of "Krebiozen," an experimental drug on the market. The man went to his doctor and begged for a Krebiozen prescription. His doctor, though suspicious of the drug, nevertheless gave it to him. Shortly afterward, the man's cancer disappeared. His doctor was astounded. The patient was ecstatic. But then the man read an article citing findings about the "ineffectiveness" of Krebiozen. Almost immediately, he had a relapse, his cancer reasserting itself with a vengeance. His doctor, by now alerted to the healing power of the man's beliefs, cleverly told his patient that the article was wrong, and that he would prescribe a new, "stronger" version of the drug that would be sure to help. It did, too. Once again the patient's condition improved. But then the almost inevitable happened: The man read of AMA and FDA findings which showed, conclusively, that Krebiozen was useless. Literally within days, the man died.

While this case underscores the almost frightening power that the mind can have, it also makes clear the large role that a doctor plays in helping to elicit the placebo response. If you trust your doctor, you're far more likely to believe in any treatment he prescribes. Therefore, the treatment is far more likely to work. The placebo effect depends on "the rapport, warmth, trust, faith, empathy or positive emotional relation-

ship between doctor and patient," Dr. Shapiro has written.

DO YOU NEED SPECIAL CARE?

One study that has conclusively shown this is a study we call the special care experiment, conducted at Massachusetts General Hospital. In this experiment, patients about to undergo surgery were divided and carefully matched according to their age, sex, the severity of their medical problem and the type of operation.

The first of the two groups was the control. An anesthesiologist visited the patients in this group before their surgery and spoke to them in a general way. He didn't discuss postoperative pain.

The patients in the second group, the "special care" group, got very different treatment. The anesthesiologist spent "quality" time with them, explaining the operation and its

The Wild, Wonderful Wart

Warts. Nobody wants them, yet medical science can't get rid of them. Burned, chopped or frozen off, "warts grow back, often in multiple clusters," writes Andrew Weil, M.D., in his book *Health and Healing*.

But what makes warts wonderful—and strange—is that *weird* treatments cure them. In fact, the weirder and wilder the treatment you try, the more likely it is to succeed. Dr. Weil, who collects wart cure stories, lists "rubbing the wart with a cut potato and burying the potato under a particular kind of tree during a likely results. He answered any of their questions. And he discussed postoperative pain with them, telling them how long it would probably last and how severe it would be.

How did the two groups compare? Not only did the people in the "special care" group require half as much pain medication as the others but they also were discharged from the hospital an average of three days earlier than the members of the other group. They had simply healed more quickly. Yet, their "special" treatment had been not medical but emotional, proving that "the essential element in all healing relationships may not be knowledge or technique, but rather care, love and concern for the patient," as Dr. Jaffe contends. And also proving that it *pays* to find a fine physician. Three days' worth of hospitalization represents a lot of money. Therefore, a doctor who cares for you and can call forth the power of your expectant faith is a doctor who could be worth his weight in at least a little gold.

But there is a problem. You see, in order for a doctor to activate the power of the placebo, he almost has to deceive us about what he is doing. How could we maintain faith in him if he were to say, "Here, I am about to give you a worthless pill"? Should we, then, hope that he'll give us a sugar pill, but say, "Here, this is a real drug. Take it and you will be cured," since he knows that his deception may help heal us? No, we shouldn't, Sissela Bok, Ph.D., a professor of philosophy at Brandeis University, told the *New York Times*. The "deception exemplified by placebos. . .carries risks not usually taken into account," she says. It "represents an inroad on informed consent, damages the institution of medicine and contributes to the erosion of confidence in medical personnel."

Even studying the placebo effect requires a breach of ethics, according to Dr. Bok. After all, there's only

particular phase of moon, selling the wart to a sibling," or "being touched by a neighborhood wart healer" among successful methods.

But warts aren't merely unlovable bumps; they're caused by viruses. So how can wild cures work, when medical ones so often don't? Dr. Weil says, "The cure may look miraculous, but it is not mystical." Quite simply, wart cures are produced by the extraordinarily potent power of *belief*. It doesn't matter that you know nothing of physiology or that you have no idea how to cure a virus. By believing in a treatment, you make it work.

"Just think what we would know if we had anything like a clear understanding of what goes on" when you make your warts wither, Lewis Thomas, M.D., one of the world's premier medical essayists, has written. We would know far more than we do about immunology, cellular biology, even about diseases like cancer and how to treat them. "Best of all, we would be finding out about a kind of superintelligence that exists in each of us. Infinitely smarter and possessed of technical knowhow far beyond our present understanding. It would be worth a War on Warts, a Conquest of Warts, a National Institute of Warts and All," Dr. Thomas feels.

one good way to study the effect: You treat one group of patients but only "pretend" to treat another, and then you see if both groups improve. Under such circumstances, you may be denying one whole group of patients medical treatment. In one controversial case, a doctor wanted to test the side effects of contraceptives. Using Mexican-American women as his subjects, he gave half of them the Pill and half of them a placebo. Since the women thought they were receiving birth control pills, one side effect of the placebo was predictable: Ten of them became pregnant. None of them had wanted to. Such experiments have helped make placebo seem a dirty word to many fine, responsible physicians.

JUST SEEING YOUR DOCTOR CAN HELP

The problem is made more complex by the fact that your doctor can act as a kind of human placebo, even when he doesn't mean at all to deceive you. Just visiting a doctor makes some people feel so much better that their illness spontaneously goes away. And if your doctor is enthusiastic about his treatment—even a treatment that turns out later to be ineffective—his or her enthusiasm is usually transmitted to you. Hopeful and happy, you are more easily healed. Of course, if your doctor starts doubting a drug, you usually sense his doubt and the drug, which may previously have been doing a perfectly fine job of healing, stops being effective. One of the lamest jokes in medicine urges doctors to "hurry up and use a treatment while it still works."

Much better advice comes from Dr. Weil. He doesn't see the ethical problem as a problem at all. The answer, he believes, is in education. Doctors need to learn just how powerful a healing tool the mind is. If placebos can work almost as well as morphine, then the mind is very powerful indeed. "Only if you imagine the mind to be unreal or unconnected to the body can you dream of ruling out the placebo effects," he says. Doctors need, in turn, to teach us how to use the powerful healing ability that we already have. Because "placebo reactions are the real meat of medicine," Dr. Weil concludes,

The Healing Relationship: Finding a Doctor You Can Believe In

The placebo effect—it tells us that the power to heal doesn't reside only in a pill, but in *us*. That if we *believe* a medicine will work, this belief somehow mobilizes a potent healing force that helps us recover. But medicine is more than pills—it's also the doctors who prescribe them. And some holistic physicians are saying that a good relationship with a doctor can also create the placebo effect.

But as we all know, good relationships are notoriously difficult to form, especially if you want to find a partner who will help you tap into the immense healing capacity within yourself. In fact, many doctors resent the implication that it is *you* doing the healing and not the pills they prescribe.

Begin your search for this person with an interview. "Make sure they have all the strong, grounded knowledge they should have, and make sure they can communicate it to you clearly," says Gregory Higgins, M.D., a doctor at the Clearlake Medical Center in Clearlake, California. "After all, they're there to provide you with technical expertise and to help you understand what's going on in your own body."

They are *not* there to be mystical miracle workers. "Doctors are just people. Make sure yours is willing to admit that," says Dr. Higgins. "Can he or she be fallible in front of you? Can he say, 'Whoops, I need to look that up'? You should have the most confidence in a doctor who can stand to be embarrassed."

For your own part, don't set a doctor

"doctors should worry about ruling them *in* rather than *out* and try to produce them more often by safe and effective means."

The "true art of medicine," says Dr. Weil, "is the ability of a practitioner to select and present to individual patients those treatments most likely to elicit healing from within [them]." The "healing art," he adds, is not found in medicines. It is found in "the secret wisdom of the body. Medicine can do no more than facilitate it."

ONLY YOU CAN HEAL

In other words, "a doctor can help, but only you can heal." Stirring words, aren't they? They're also hopeful words. But let's face it, they're not, from a practical standpoint, very helpful words. Not many of us can turn on our healing powers like a light bulb; most of us are still wondering if there's a switch. How, then, do we learn to trust in and control our own healing?

First of all, we should feel confident. As Dr. Jaffe says reassuringly, "You have much greater con-trol over your own destiny than you probably realize." Remember that the placebo effect doesn't depend "on something that doctors do to you. Healing doesn't happen outside of your own self. Once you begin to overcome your feelings of helplessness, you're on your way to becoming your own healer," he says.

To do this, we need to "see healing as an innate capacity of the body rather than something to be sought outside it," Dr. Weil says. We must understand just how closely the body and the mind are bound together. If the evidence for the immense power of the placebo hasn't already convinced you, consider this: When the movie *Lawrence of Arabia* was first shown in theaters, the concession stands were swamped at intermissions with people begging for liquids of any kind. Sales were far, far above normal. Why? People were watching parched landscape after parched landscape on the screen and their minds were saying "thirst." Their bodies responded, though there was no "real" reason for their thirst. Lawrence might be marching across the desert; they were sitting in humidified theaters.

up to fail. "You can't just sit back and say 'cure me,'" Dr. Higgins says. "It's very easy for a doctor to look medical and correct and to smile at the right time. It's not easy to heal."

What you must recognize, he continues, is that "the level of responsibility that a patient holds a doctor accountable for determines the level of treatment the doctor gives. The more helpless you as a patient are, the more you throw yourself on a doctor's mercy, demanding some kind of healing miracle, the less responsibility you call forth from your doctor. I know that from my own practice. If I have a patient come in who can knowledgeably explain what he expects of me, I naturally respond with greater sympathy," and an increased sense of how healing is, at its best, a process of *inter*action between doctor and patient.

"Healing is not something that's done *to* you, but something that's done *with* you," Dr. Higgins says. The difference is something like the difference between a dependent child's relationship to his parents versus an intelligent adult's relationship to another intelligent adult. It is not a relationship of dependence but of mutual aid. "Healing is a process of growth and change in whatever form and it's not always pleasant," Dr. Higgins concludes. "I know it's not easy, but what the healing process ultimately requires from both the healer and the patient is. . .maturity."

An even more remarkable instance of the power of the mind is evident in "pseudocyesis," or false pregnancy. Women who want desperately to be pregnant may convince themselves that they are. They stop having periods, their breasts and belly swell and they generally have all the symptoms of approaching motherhood. Doctors have even diagnosed them as pregnant. Sometimes they go into false labor. And one memorable case—complete with all symptoms—has been reported in a male. All of this when there never was any fetus. When all there was, was an idea.

The power of an idea allowed psychologist Rollo May, Ph.D., to overcome life-threatening tuberculosis, he believes. "After becoming aware of my body and its disease, I began to get better. I. . .invented a sort of meditation for myself, which was a capacity to actually sense what was happening in my own body," he says.

This is exactly the strategy that leading physicians and psychiatrists recommend you adopt in order to heal yourself. "You need to learn to treat your body as you would anyone with whom you share a meaningful relationship," Dr. Jaffe, a leader in holistic health care, says. "To communicate with someone you care for in the outside world, you have to use language. Well, we want to estab-

Fire Walking Is a Hot Idea

Feets afire! If you fear that would happen should you try walking across a bed of burning coals, fear not. In fact, learning to "transform fear into power" is just what fire walking is all about, according to Eric Best, Ph.D., head of the Institute for Science and Humanism in El Segundo, California. Dr. Best, who has taught hundreds of people to fire walk in his 4½-hour seminars, begins each with lessons in "clearing a space inside you, psychologically socially, physically. Then I try to take that opening and literally fill it with new energy."

If that sounds a little ethereal, what happens next convinces everyone that Dr. Best's feet are actually planted firmly on the ground—and are remarkably heat resistant as well: He walks across 500- to 1,000-degree coals. Typically, 75 to 80 percent of the seminar participants—ordinary people ranging from businessmen to the unemployed—follow him. Burning coals, bare feet and no blisters? How? "The big secret is really no secret at all," Dr. Best says. "If you *believe* that you can, you can." Even for those who only watch, the seminars are beneficial. "People have so much fear, and I don't mean just the big, specific fears, like of death or of cancer," Dr. Best explains. "I mean our day-to-day fears, such as whether we can say what we think and still be liked or whether we dare look for a better job and risk losing the one we have. The quality of our life suffers because of all these 'little capitulations.'"

Fire walking can help you reverse that. "When people realize that this big fear they have, of the coals burning them, isn't necessarily realistic, when they recognize that they *themselves* control their physical reality, then their whole internal point of view sort of shifts. They think, gee whiz, if I can do that, I don't need to be afraid of my boss or of looking silly or whatever. It's a tremendous feeling."

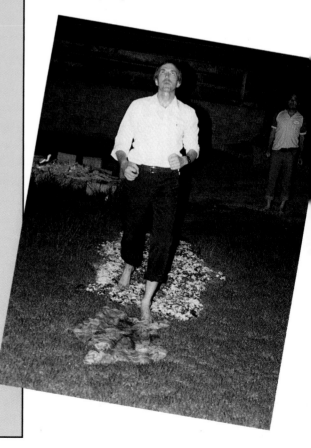

lish the same kind of communication with our own bodies." This is by no means a simple task. "You can't just say, 'Hey, body, be healed,'" Dr. Jaffee explains. You have to learn the right language.

IMAGINE YOUR ILLS AWAY

In Dr. Jaffe's view, this language is the language of imagery. "The whole relationship we have to our bodies is a little like the relationship that most of us have to computers. Many of us don't understand microchips or any of the more technical components of a computer or really how it works. But we don't need to. We can still use the software. It's in a language we can understand. Imaging is like software for our bodies."

It is the most useful self-healing technique because "our bodies respond to pictures when they don't or can't respond to words," Dr. Jaffe says. "In imaging, you create a picture or a felt sense of what you want to have happen and of how you want the body to move toward that. For example, if you want to lower your blood pressure, you need to talk your blood vessels into relaxing. So you might try imagining little tubes becoming ever more flexible, more elastic, allowing more liquid to flow through them more easily. Any similar images will do. It really doesn't matter whether your mental image is fanciful or technical or whatever you feel most comfortable creating. The important thing is that you feel, deep inside your own body, that you are communicating with yourself."

"Communicate with yourself" is also Dr. Benson's prescription for healing. "Our brains are tremendously complex and have great potential for triggering dramatic reactions" in our bodies, he says. But we must carefully create the right atmosphere and attitudes for our healing. The author of *The Relaxation Response* and *Beyond the Relaxation Response,* Dr. Benson, not surprisingly, advocates relaxation as the means for bridging any gap between mind and body. But his relaxation is not so simple as a nap or a few quiet moments in front of the television.

Is Pot a Placebo?

When someone says "hallucinogen," do you think instantly of horrid opium dens where yellowed, emaciated youths loll about in various stages of dissipation? Or do you imagine more pleasant parties, with glittering-eyed sophisticates staring at each other, discovering they suddenly know most of the secrets of the universe? Well, instead of either of these, you could—but probably didn't—think "placebo." Andrew Weil, M.D., author of *The Natural Mind,* thinks you should. He believes the characteristic effects of mind-altering drugs are largely in the mind. "To my mind," he says, "the best term for marijuana is 'active placebo.'"

Of course, since use of these drugs is illegal, studies of them in use have been fairly scarce. But of these, many have produced almost "mind-altering" findings in support of Dr. Weil's view. For example, a 1971 study showed that a placebo can, in some cases, make you more "high" than marijuana. In the experiment, regular users of the drug were asked to smoke several very potent varieties, a somewhat less potent one and, finally, a placebo, and then to rate how "high" each substance made them feel. While the people involved reported the greatest effect from the very strong marijuana, they felt "higher" after smoking the placebo than they felt after smoking the weaker marijuana. Therefore, the researchers concluded, below a certain strength, marijuana's effects may depend on psychology and not pharmacology.

Amazingly, very potent hallucinogens, including LSD, have also been proven to depend on a placebo effect. In one famous study, volunteers were told they were about to be given LSD. Actually, they were given tap water. But when they were then asked about the symptoms this "drug" produced, many of them reported at least some of the reactions that can result from LSD use, including drowsiness, sweaty palms and a feeling of dreaminess. Pretty potent stuff, that tap water.

These experiments help to account for the huge variations in people's responses to hallucinogens. But the real lesson to be gleaned from the drug studies, Dr. Weil stresses, is that being "high" is, at bottom, a state of mind. *You* produce it, independent of the drug. The drug is just a crutch, a placebo.

"Each patient carries his own doctor inside him. They come to us not knowing that truth. We are at our best when we give the doctor who resides within each patient a chance to go to work."

—Dr. Albert Schweitzer

It is closer to what Dr. Weil recommends when he says that there is "great value in learning to relax, not in the usual, superficial ways, but in the profound way that reveals our true capacities and strengths."

RELAX: HEALING IS NOT SO HARD

The road to "profound" relaxation—and healing—begins with four fairly straightforward steps, Dr. Benson believes. This constitutes the "technique" necessary for relaxation:

1. Find a quiet place. You need to "turn off" external distractions.

2. Focus on an object. Concentrating on a particular sound or symbol will help eliminate distracting thoughts.

3. Maintain a passive attitude. Try to empty your mind of internal distractions.

4. Get into a comfortable position.

The "heart" of therapeutic relaxation, though, is in replenishing your emptied mind with *belief. Strong belief.* "If you truly believe in your personal philosophy or religious faith—if you are committed, mind and soul, to your world view—you may well be capable of achieving remarkable feats of mind and body," Dr. Benson maintains. He doesn't suggest you believe in any one particular philosophy or religion. But it is essential that you believe strongly in *something*. Belief in yourself and your ability to cooperate with and heal your body is a good starting point. Then, in selecting a word, phrase or mental picture for Step 2, choose one that somehow exemplifies your belief and concentrate all your mental energy on this. Doing so will help you to activate the power of "personal belief to heal a very large variety of physical maladies," Dr. Benson says. It can help us especially well to overcome those "problems that we have tried to treat only through physical means or, perhaps, have regarded as medically untreatable."

What relaxation most demands from you is that you "turn your attention inward," which "is my first advice to patients," Dr. Jaffe says.

You simply can't initiate self-healing if you don't listen to your body. "The placebo effect in action is a two-way process!" Dr. Jaffe insists. "Your saying, 'Hey, body, shape up,' represents only half of the relationship. In the other half, you must find out *why* things went wrong in the first place. If you're getting headaches because you hate your work, then accusing your body of causing you headaches won't get rid of your pain. You need to examine your life and try to see what led to the breakdown in the first place. Try to understand what your body is telling you before you tell your body what to do."

A considerate, caring and reciprocating relationship between your mind and your body, then, is the foundation of all health and healing. "This is what makes your self-healing so much more powerful than when you rely fully on some doctor. He may pat you on the head and say, 'Get well,' and you may. Temporarily. But only *you* can listen to your body and make changes. You're the only one who can hear what your body has to say," Dr. Jaffe concludes.

You're the only one, ultimately, who can heal you. This is not exactly a new insight. Over a century ago, the great British physician Sir William Osler told his students:

"Ask not what kind of illness the patient has, ask what kind of patient has the illness."

If you read between the lines, he said:

"A patient's mind, his emotions can cause his illness; by extension, surely, they can promote his health."

Sir William was about a century ahead of his time. Only now are large numbers of doctors beginning to share his view. But Sir William didn't go far enough. With what we now know of the immense powers waiting for us in our own minds, we would say something less lyrical, maybe, but more uplifting, like:

"Ask not what kind of illness you have. Ask not even what you can do against your illness.

Instead—ask not at all. Listen and take responsibility for your own illness and then 'put your mind' to doing what is needed to fight against it."

The strongest medicine of all is you.

Source Notes

Chapter 1

Page 4

"Drug Companies Pocket Top Profits" adapted from "The 500: The Fortune Directory of the Largest U.S. Industrial Corporations," *Fortune*, April 30, 1984.

Pages 6-7

Map adapted from "Medical Detective Story: A Polio Virus Tracked Down," by Harold M. Schmeck, Jr., *New York Times*, August 28, 1979.

Chapter 5

Pages 80-81

"Dangerous Herbs" adapted from *Herbal Medications*, by David G. Spoerke, Jr. (Santa Barbara, Calif., Woodbridge, 1980)
and
The Honest Herbal, by Varro E. Tyler (Philadelphia: George F. Stickley, 1982)
and
Herbs That Heal, by William A. R. Thomson (New York: Charles Scribner's Sons, 1976)
and
The Encyclopedia of Herbs and Herbalism, Malcolm Stuart, ed. (New York: Grosset & Dunlap, 1979)
and
"Plants That Bring Health—or Death," by John Humphreys, *New Scientist*, February 25, 1982
and
Poisonous Plants of the United States and Canada, by John M. Kingsbury (Englewood Cliffs, N.J., Prentice-Hall, 1964)
and
Healing Plants: A Modern Herbal, William A. R. Thomson, ed. (United Kingdom: McGraw-Hill, 1978).

Chapter 6

Page 87

"The Best Method for You" adapted from *Contraception: Comparing the Options*, by the Department of Health and Human Services, U.S. Food and Drug Administration (Washington, D.C.: Department of Health and Human Services, 1980)
and
Population Bulletin: Understanding U.S. Fertility: Findings from the National Survey of Family Growth, Cycle III, by William F. Pratt, William D. Mosher, Christine A. Bachrach and Marjorie C. Horn (Washington, D.C.: Population Reference Bureau, 1984)
and
The Birth Control Book, by Howard I. Shapiro (New York: St. Martin's, 1977)
and
Making Choices: Evaluating the Health Risks and Benefits of Birth Control Methods, by Howard W. Ory, Jacqueline Darroch Forrest and Richard Lincoln (Washington, D.C.: The Alan Guttmacher Institute, 1983)
and
My Body, My Health, by Felicia Hance Stewart, Gary K. Stewart, Felicia Jane Guest and Robert A. Hatcher (New York: Bantam Books, 1981)
and
Every Woman's Pharmacy: A Guide to Safe Drug Use, by William F. Rayburn, Frederick P. Zuspan and Jeanne Tashian Fitzgerald (St. Louis: C. V. Mosby, 1983).

Chapter 7

Pages 106-117

"Drug Side Effects" adapted from *Physicians' Desk Reference*, 38th ed. (Oradell, N.J.: Medical Economics Co., 1984)
and
The Essential Guide to Prescription Drugs, 3d ed., by James M. Long (New York: Harper & Row, 1982)
and
Complete Guide to Prescription and Non-Prescription Drugs, by H. Winter Griffith (Tucson, Ariz.: HPBooks, 1983)
and
Food and Medication Interactions, 4th ed., by Dorothy E. Powers and Ann O. Moore (Tempe, Ariz.: F-M I Publishing, 1983)
and
The Physicians' Drug Manual, Rubin Bressler, Morton D. Bogdonoff and Genell J. Subak-Sharpe, eds. (Garden City, N.Y.: Doubleday, 1981)
and
Hazards of Medication, 2d ed., by Eric W. Martin (Philadelphia: J.B. Lippincott, 1978).

Chapter 7

Pages 118-119

"Possible Sexual Side Effects" adapted from *Physicians' Desk Reference*, 38th ed. (Oradell, N.J.: Medical Economics Co., 1984).

Illustration Credits

Bascove: pp. 2; 39; 44; 67; 123; 125; 129; 131; 133; 135; 137; 141; 143; 145. Lisa Gatti: pp. viii-1. Susan Gray: pp. 4; 76; 157. Jerry O'Brien: p. 148. Mary Anne Shea: pp. 6-7; 45; 59; 88. Wendy Wray: p. 132.

Photography Credits

Cover: Angelo M. Caggiano.
Staff Photographers—Angelo M. Caggiano: pp. 102-103. Carl Doney: pp. 56-57; 87. T. L. Gettings: p. 72. John P. Hamel: pp. 22-23; 146-147. Mark Lenny: pp. 53; 66. Alison Miksch: pp. 18-19; 21; 30-31; 70-71; 82-83; 155. Margaret Skrovanek: pp. 42-43; 69; 92; 98-99; 120-121; 157. Christie C. Tito: pp. 46; 48-49; 78-79; 152.

Other Photographers—Morton Beebe/The Image Bank: p. 149. Lawrence Fried/The Image Bank: p. 61. M. Martin/The Image Bank: p. 8.

Additional Photographs Courtesy of—Eric N. Best, Ph.D./The Institute For Science and Humanism, El Segundo, Calif.: p. 160. The Bettman Archive: pp. 16; 46-47; 150.

Special Thanks to—Eric Best, Ph.D., Institute for Science and Humanism, El Segundo, Calif.; Carolina Biological Supply, Burlington, N.C.; Continental Galleries, Allentown, Pa.; Coopersburg Pharmacy, Coopersburg, Pa.; Dorneyville Pharmacy, Dorneyville, Pa.; Rea & Derick, Allentown, Pa.

Index

Rodale Press, Inc., publishes PREVENTION®, the better health magazine.
For information on how to order your subscription,
write to PREVENTION®, Emmaus, PA 18049.